Evidence-Based Clinical Gastroenterology

John Libbey Eurotext
127, avenue de la République
92120 Montrouge
Tél. : 01 46 73 06 60

John Libbey and Company Ltd
13, Smiths Yard, Summerley Street
London SW18 4HR, England
Tel. : 1 947 27 77

John Libbey CIC
Via L. Spallanzani, 11
00161, Rome, Italie
Tel. : 06 862 289

© John Libbey Eurotext, 1997
ISBN : 2-7420-0192-1

Il est interdit de reproduire intégralement ou partiellement le présent ouvrage - loi du 11 mars 1957 - sans autorisation de l'éditeur ou du Centre Français du Copyright, 6 *bis*, rue Gabriel-Laumain, 75010 Paris, France.

Evidence-Based Clinical Gastroenterology

Edited by
M.J.G. Farthing
J.J. Misiewicz

Postgraduate Course 1997
Birmingham, October 19

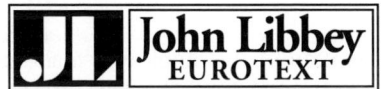

The publication of this book was made possible
thanks to the support from the Takeda Laboratories

Contents

List of contributors VII

Foreword
M.J.G. Farthing, J.J. Misiewicz.. IX

***Helicobacter pylori* infection and gastric cancer risk**
G.N.J. Tytgat... 1

Inoperable oesophageal cancer
R. Lambert.. 9

Treatment of intractable reflux
J. Janssens.. 15

Causes and consequences of intestinal failure: the model of the short bowel
B. Messing.. 27

Management of primary biliary cirrhosis
P.L.M. Jansen... 41

Hepatitis C: current concepts
G.M. Dusheiko.. 55

Outcome of surgery for colitis
N.S. Williams.. 69

Management of pain in chronic pancreatitis
P.U. Reber, M.W. Büchler.. 81

Management of "anismus" in adults
M.A. Kamm... 95

List of contributors

Büchler M.W., Department of Visceral and Transplantation Surgery, Universitätsspital Bern, CH-3010 Bern, Switzerland.

Dusheiko G.M., Royal Free Hospital and School of Medicine, Pond Street, Hampstead NW3 2QG, United Kingdom.

Jansen P.L.M., Department of Gastroenterology and Hepatology, University Hospital Groningen, PO Box 30.001, 9700 RB Groningen, The Netherlands.

Janssens J., Center for Gastroenterological Research, Faculty of Medicine, Department of Pathophysiology, K.U. Leuven, Herestraat 49, 3000 Leuven, Belgium.

Kamm M.A., Physiology Unit, St Mark's Hospital, Northwick Park, Watford Road, Harrow, Middlesex HAI 3UJ, United Kingdom.

Lambert R., Department of Digestive Diseases, Hôpital Édouard-Herriot, Place d'Arsonval, 69437 Lyon Cedex 03, France.

Messing B., Service d'Hépato-Gastroentérologie, Hôpital Saint-Lazare, 107 bis, rue du Faubourg-Saint-Denis, 75475 Paris Cedex 10, France.

Reber P.U., Department of Visceral and Transplantation Surgery, Universitätsspital Bern, CH-3010 Bern, Switzerland.

Tytgat G.N.J., Department of Gastroenterology-Hepatology, Academic Medical Center, University of Amsterdam, PO Box 22700, 1100 DE Amsterdam, The Netherlands.

Williams N.S., Academic Department of Surgery, The Royal London Hospital, Whitechapel, London E1 1BB, United Kingdom.

Foreword

During the past five years evidence-based medicine has become the *sine qua non* of clinical practice. Extremists would insist that treatment could only be offered to a patient providing there is irrefutable evidence that it works. Randomised controlled trials and high quality meta-analyses have assumed a prominent position unrivalled by other tools of human investigation. Many clinicians, however, have been attempting to treat their patients on the basis of published evidence for many decades and the ascendancy of this new dictum came as a surprise to some and perhaps was slightly insulting to others. Nevertheless, it must be conceded that there has been widespread, inappropriate use of many treatments in clinical practice both medical and surgical. "Clinical experience" and anecdote have driven the practice of many clinicians, often resulting in the use of ineffective treatments and on occasions putting patients at the risk of adverse effects of therapy which has no proven clinical benefit. Thus, the rise of evidence-based medicine has re-emphasised the need for high quality evidence that management interventions will actually benefit our patients, a therapeutic goal which becomes increasingly important as treatments become more expensive and carry high risks.

Unfortunately, evidence-based medicine is not a panacea. All clinicians will recognize clinical problems for which the evidence is just not available or is of such poor quality that it cannot be accepted with any confidence. We have tried to explore some of these areas in the European Association of Gastroenterology and Endoscopy Postgraduate Course held in Birmingham, October 1997, the proceedings of which are summarized in this book. The topics we chose are common problems in clinical gastroenterological practice, but for which clear evidence on the appropriate management strategy is either incomplete or absent. We have chosen experts in the field to trawl up what evidence there is and to underscore the management questions that still need to be answered. Perhaps we should have called the course "Non evidence-based gastroenterology"!

Michael Farthing
George Misiewicz
October 1997

Helicobacter pylori infection and gastric cancer risk

G.N.J. Tytgat

Academic Medical Center, Department of Gastroenterology-Hepatology, Amsterdam, The Netherlands

Summary

H. pylori *is a leading factor in the multistep process that ultimately leads to gastric cancer. The evidence has been summarized in several overviews. Acquisition of the infection early in life increases the late gastric cancer risk. A conservative estimate would indicate that approximately 30% of gastric cancers in the developed world and 50% in the developing world may be attributable to* H. pylori *infection. Goldstone and Dixon have summarized schematically the sequence of phenotypic and genotypic changes that ultimately lead to intestinal type of gastric cancer whereas Solcia et al. have compared intestinal and diffuse type of gastric cancer. Development of atrophic gastritis is likely to be a dominant step in the process leading to intestinal type of gastric carcinoma.*

H. pylori is a leading factor in the multistep process that ultimately leads to gastric cancer. The evidence has been summarized in several overviews [1, 2]. Acquisition of the infection early in life increases the late gastric cancer risk [3]. A conservative estimate would indicate that approximately 30% of gastric cancers in the developed world and 50% in the developing world may be attributable to *H. pylori* infection [4].

Goldstone and Dixon [5] have summarized schematically the sequence of phenotypic and genotypic changes that ultimately lead to intestinal type of gastric cancer (summarized in *figure 1*) whereas Solcia *et al.* [6] have compared intestinal and diffuse type of gastric cancer (summarized in *figure 2*). Development of atrophic gastritis is likely to be a dominant step in the process leading to intestinal type of gastric carcinoma [7].

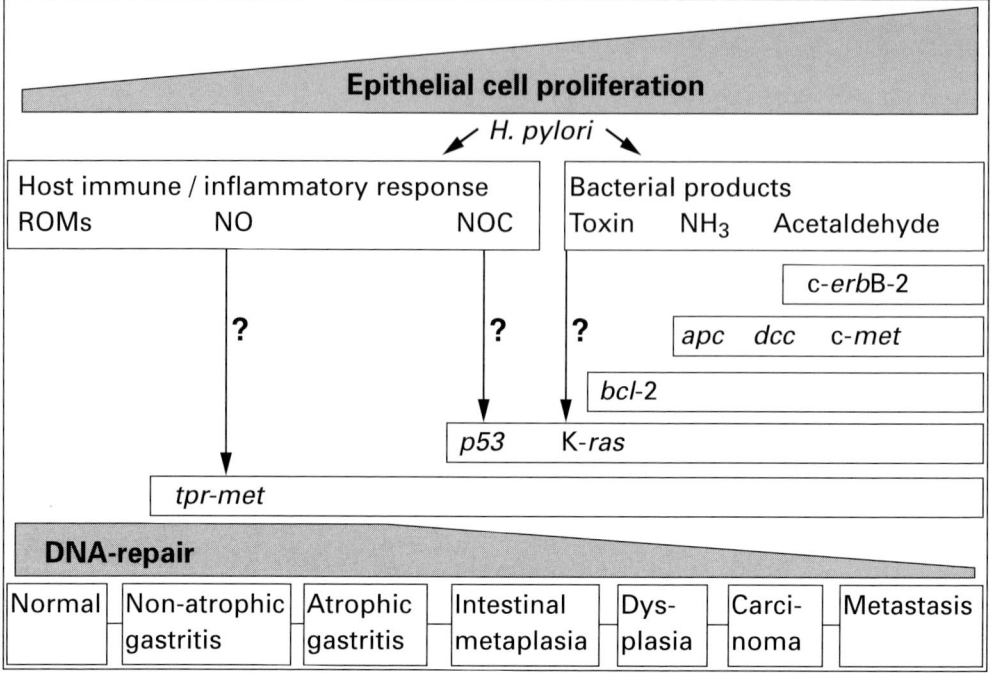

Figure 1. Schematic overview of the putative sequence of changes leading to gastric adenocarcinoma of the intestinal type, malignancy according to Goldstone, Quirke and Dixon [5].

The point of "no return" in the multistep carcinogenic process

Treatment of *H. pylori* infected individuals would obviously be of no benefit if detection of at risk individuals would occur beyond a point of "no return", where the development of malignancy would progress in an unrelenting fashion despite cure of the infection. This point of "no return", if it exists, is unknown *(figure 3)*. In my perception, the point of "no return" is passed once there is sufficient atrophy of the mucosa to interfere with intragastric acidity. The ensuing a- or hypochlorhydria will then allow overgrowth of bacteria, both aerobes and anaerobes. These bacteria have reductases that convert nitrate into nitrite with the potential to generate N-nitroso compounds even at high gastric pH [8]. These individuals also have low concentrations of ascorbic acid in gastric juice [9]. Loss of this powerful anti-oxidant favours nitrite and nitrosamine formation [10] and reduces scavenging of mucosal oxygen radicals [11].

Others question the existence of a "no-return" point and postulate that, as inflammation is ongoing, arrest or reversibility of the carcinogenic pathway might be possible through abolition of the cell damaging and mutagenic inflammatory mediators, such as nitric oxide and other oxygen radicals capable of inducing mutations of DNA [12].

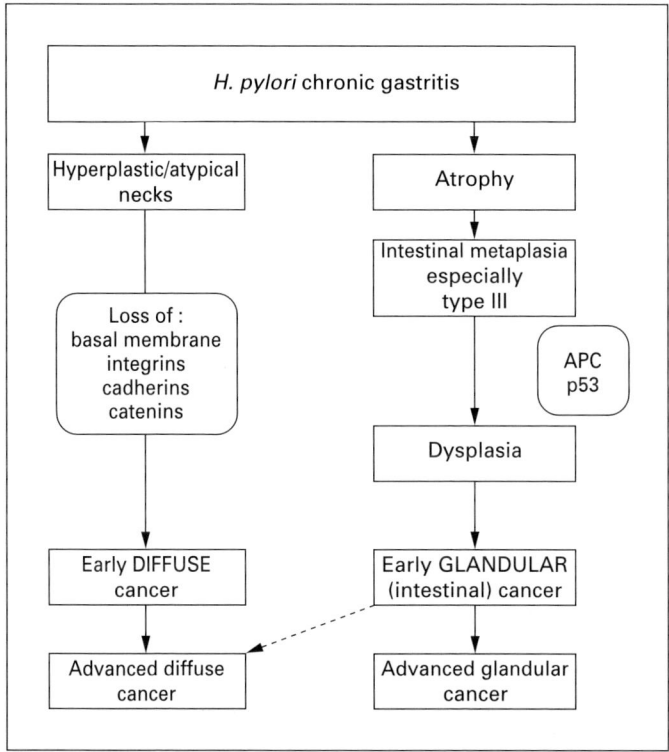

Figure 2. Schematic overview of the putative sequence of changes leading to intestinal and diffuse gastric cancer according to Solcia et al. [6].

Reversibility of gastric atrophy and intestinal metaplasia

Atrophic gastritis and intestinal metaplasia are well recognized precancerous lesions. Potential reversibility of atrophic changes and intestinal metaplasia after *H. pylori* cure would theoretically be of immense importance. Data on reversibility are limited and somewhat conflicting as summarized in *table I*. Although the data are still limited, it would appear that some reversibility of atrophy is possible. Whether full blown extensive intestinal metaplasia is reversible, is still a debatable point.

Gastric cancer prevention through *H. pylori* eradication

Proof that *H. pylori* cure decreases gastric cancer risk is lacking. No well controlled prospective studies have been carried out so far to shed some light upon this question.

In a randomized study of early cancer in Japan [13], patients with early gastric cancer who were positive for *H. pylori* were divided after endoscopic therapy of the index ma-

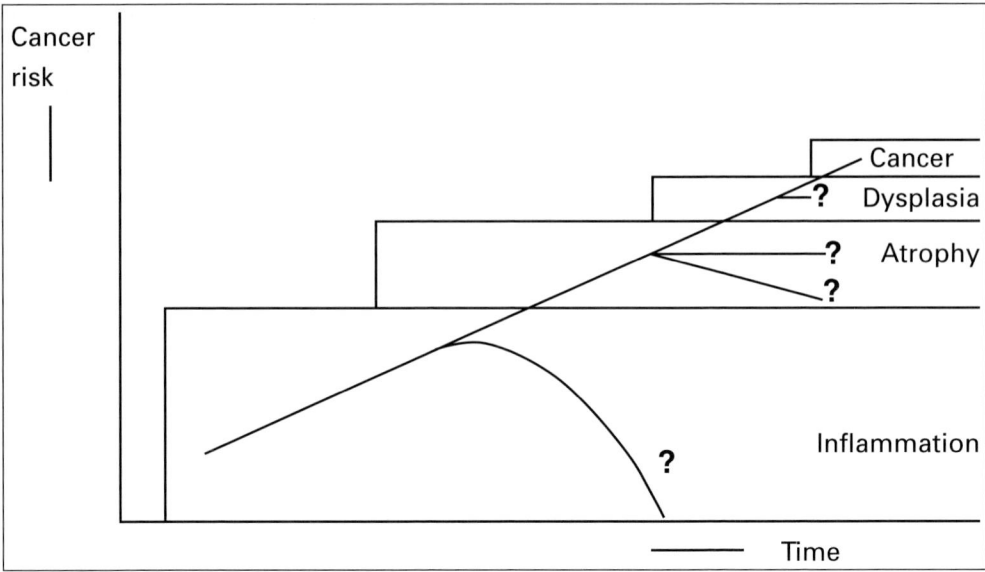

Figure 3. Hypothetical positioning of the point of "no-return".

Table I. Evolution of gastric atrophy and intestinal metaplasia scores after *H. pylori* cure

	n	Atrophy score before	Atrophy score after	Average follow-up	Intestinal metaplasia score before	Intestinal metaplasia score after	Average follow-up
Genta [23]	11				A 16 C 5.0	A 13 C 2.6	1 year 1 year
Cayla [24]	28	1.2	0.9	5 years	1.0	0.3	5 years
Haruma [25]	20				A 1.7 C 1.4	A 1.4 C 0.9	6 months 6 months
Satoh [26]	23	A 1.3 C 0.0	A 0.9 C 0.0	29 months 29 months	A 0.9 C 0.1	A 0.8 C 0.0	29 months 29 months
Van der Hulst [27]	150	A* 1.6 A** 0.8	A* 1.6 A** 0.7	1 year 1 year	A* 0.9 A** 0.2	A* 1.0 A** 0.2	1 year 1 year
Van der Hulst [28]	140	A 2.0	A 1.4	4 years	A 0.8	A 0.7	4 years

A = antrum; C = corpus; A* = cagA pos.; A** = cagA neg.

lignancy into 2 treatment groups: one group received *H. pylori* eradication therapy and the other did not. In the group who underwent eradication treatment no metachronous new cancers developed, whereas in the *H. pylori* positive group, 6 (9%) new cancers developed.

In a Swedish study of hip replacement patients [14], it was found that patients had a reduced risk of gastric cancer during follow-up. The authors suggested that the antibiotics given to such patients in connection with the hip surgery might have cured the *H. pylori* infection, thereby reducing the ultimate cancer risk.

Obviously many more detailed studies are necessary to fully answer the above question on cancer prevention through *H. pylori* cure. Several such studies are underway in China and the results are to be expected a few years from now. Another cancer prevention trial in Europe is years, if not decades from completion [15].

Preventive screening and treatment of infected individuals

Screening strategies have been suggested to identify and treat infected individuals. In Asia, screening 100,00 people aged 55 would be expected to identify about 80,000 individuals who are *H. pylori* infected of whom 6,400 might develop cancer. In a European country, only 1,600 cancer cases would be expected in a similar sample. Those in favour of screening and subsequent treatment would argue that it is cheap and reliable. *H. pylori* is the only treatable infectious disease with a high rate of morbidity and mortality that is not subject of an all out programme to eradicate it from the population. Those against would stress the risks involved and the potential of inducing antimicrobial resistance. Resistance to clarithromycin and metronidazole is possible in a large proportion of those that fail eradication therapy. This phenomenon together with the rapidly rising primary metronidazole and clarithromycin resistance might seriously jeopardize the overall usefulness of an intervention strategy. Moreover there are the risks of poly-antimicrobial therapy and the even occasional mortality due to pseudomembranous colitis. But most importantly, it is not known at what stage the progression to cancer becomes irreversible. One therefore does not know the age at which intervention might be successful. Moreover population screening poses ethical problems, specially when screening and treatment engender undue anxiety, or serious adverse events in apparently healthy individuals.

An alternative approach is what has been called "opportunistic screening" where testing occurs after the patient contacts a medical practitioner about a specific complaint. Patients with dyspepsia could as a rule be tested and treated for *H. pylori* infection. This policy might prevent gastric cancer in an individual patient, although it is unlikely to have a substantial impact on the overall gastric cancer load, because only a small proportion of at risk patients will attend with dyspeptic symptoms well before overt malignancy develops.

Preventive screening and treatment of subgroups at excessively enhanced high cancer risk

If screening all asymptomatic individuals is considered inappropriate, one might perhaps consider selecting individuals of known enhanced cancer risk. Well known epidemiological risk factors are: (1) early acquisition of *H. pylori*; (2) low socioeconomic class and background; (3) diet low in anti-oxidants; (4) blood group A; (5) familial occurrence of gastric cancer [16]; (6) certain HLA-associations [17], (7) CagA positivity; (8) atrophic gastritis; (9) a(hypo)gammaglobulinaemia [18].

Based upon the previously well documented association between a- or hypochlorhydria and gastric cancer, the subgroup of patients with a- or hypochlorhydria due to *H. pylori*-induced corpus gastritis and atrophy is likely to contain the association between infection and cancer. The ability to identify this subgroup should be important, as it would allow it to be targeted for *H. pylori* eradication therapy. Pepsinogen 1 or pepsinogen 1/2 ratio could be a useful marker to select those patients at enhanced risk [19, 20].

Patients with agammaglobulinaemia with compromised immune surveillance also run a higher risk of development of atrophy and cancer [21].

Concluding remarks

The pathogenic mechanisms reviewed and summarized by Goldstone and Dixon, and summarized in *figure 1* offer a plausible explanation for the role of *H. pylori* in the initiation and promotion of gastric cancer. Others have used epidemiological data to conclude that *H. pylori* is carcinogenic. Considering the universality of *H. pylori* infection and its attributable risk in cancer causation, the public health implications are profound. However it is by no means obvious what measures could and should be taken to aid cancer prevention.

Possibilities include education as to hygiene which could help to prevent person-to-person bacterial spread, and education as to nutrition. More radical forms of intervention could include population-based eradication therapy, or anti-*H. pylori* vaccination.

Given the current costs of effective antimicrobial treatment, difficulties with compliance, the possibility of side-effects and induction of resistance, the potential for re-infection in high-incidence countries, mass eradication programmes are in all probability impractical.

The development of a vaccine appears to offer the best hope for the elimination of the infection, but a useful vaccine is probably at least 10 years away from clinical applicability.

More evidence to prove the cause may only come through intervention studies. While intervention studies have great merit, they will take years to complete and may be technically impractical.

If large scale population-based intervention trials are impractical or not realistic at present, physicians should seriously consider screening and treatment when approached by individual asymptomatic patients under the following circumstances:
– asymptomatic first-degree relatives of gastric cancer patients;
– individuals with established atrophic gastritis with/without intestinal metaplasia; the risk for gastric cancer may be elevated up to 90-fold in subjects with severe atrophic pangastritis [22];
– individuals with (hypo)achlorhydria;
– individuals in need for long-term suppression of gastric acidity; this topic is at present considered highly controversial. Yet, amalgamation of all available evidence points pro-

bably to accelerated development of mucosal atrophy, in the presence of long-term suppression of intragastric acidity in *H. pylori* infected patients;
- individuals with immunodeficiency;
- individuals with ethnic risk factors;
- individuals with strong wish to be tested and treated.

References

1. Correa P. *Helicobacter pylori* and gastric carcinogenesis. *Am J Surg Pathol* 1995; 19 (Suppl 1): S37-S43.
2. Forman D, Webb P, Parsonnet J. *Helicobacter pylori* and gastric cancer. *Lancet* 1994; 343: 243-4.
3. Blaser MJ, Chyou PH, Nomura A. Age at establishment of *Helicobacter pylori* infection and gastric carcinoma, gastric ulcer, and duodenal ulcer risk. *Cancer Res* 1995; 55: 562-5.
4. Forman D. *Helicobacter pylori* and gastric cancer. *Scand J Gastroenterol* 1996; 31 (Suppl 220): 23-6.
5. Goldstone AR, Quirke Ph, Dixon MF. *Helicobacter pylori* infection and gastric cancer. *J Pathol* 1996; 179: 129-37.
6. Solcia E, Fiocca R, Luinetti O, Villani L, Padovan L, Calistri D, Ranzani GN, Chiaravalli A, Capella C. Intestinal and diffuse gastric cancers arise in a different background of *Helicobacter pylori* gastritis through different gene involvement. *Am J Surg Pathol* 1996; 20 (Suppl 1): S8-S22.
7. Hansson LE, Nyrén O, Hsing AW, Bergström R, Josefsson S, Chow WH, Fraumeni JF, Adami HO. The risk of stomach cancer in patients with gastric or duodenal ulcer disease. *N Engl J Med* 1996; 335: 242-9.
8. Keefer LK, Roller PP. N-nitrosation by nitrite ion in neutral and basal medium. *Science* 1973; 181: 1245-7.
9. Ruiz B, Rood JC, Fontham ETH, et al. Vitamin C concentration in gastric juice before and after anti-*Helicobacter pylori* treatment. *Am J Gastroenterol* 1994; 89: 533-9.
10. Carton Rood J, Ruiz B, Fontham ETH, Malcom GT, Hunter FM, Sobhan M, Johnson WD, Correa P. *Helicobacter pylori*-associated gastritis and the ascorbic acid concentration in gastric juice. *Nutr Cancer* 1994; 22: 65-72.
11. Drake IM, Davies MJ, Mapstone NP, Dixon MF, Schorah CJ, White KLM, Chalmers DM, Axon ATR. Ascorbic acid may protect against human gastric cancer by scavenging mucosal oxygen radicals. *Carcinogenesis* 1996; 17: 559-62.
12. Nguyen T, Brunson D, Crespi J, et al. DNA damage and mutations in human cells exposed to nitric oxide *in vitro*. *Proc Natl Acad Sci USA* 1992; 89: 303-9.
13. Uemura N, Mukai T, Okamoto S, Yamaguchi S, Mashiba H, Taniyama K, Sasaki N, Haruma K, Sumii K, Kajiyama G. *Helicobacter pylori* eradication inhibits the growth of intestinal type of gastric cancer in initial stage. *Gastroenterology* 1996; 110: A282.
14. Nyrén O. Personal communication.
15. Reed PI, Johnston BJ. Prévention primaire du cancer gastrique. L'étude d'intervention ECP-MI; Primary prevention of gastric cancer – The ECP-IM intervention study. *Acta Endoscopica* 1995; 25: 45-54.
16. Kokkola A, Valle J, Haapiainen R, Sipponen P, Kivilaakso E, Puolakkainen P. *Helicobacter pylori* infection in young patients with gastric carcinoma. *Scand J Gastroenterol* 1996; 31: 643-7.
17. Lee JE, Lowy AM, Thompson WA, Lu M, Loflin PT, Skibber JM, Evans DB, Curley SA, Menasfield PF, Reveille JD. Association of gastric adenocarcinoma with the HLA class II gene DQB1*0301. *Gastroenterology* 1996; 111: 426-32.
18. Fuchs CS, Mayer RJ. Gastric carcinoma. *N Engl J Med* 1995; 333: 32-41.

staging of the morphology and depth of the tumour is completed by echoendoscopy and computed tomography (mediastinal and abdominal) for the detection of liver or pulmonary metastases. The evaluation concerns curative or palliative resection, according to the prediction of complete or incomplete removal of all tumour tissue. If performed, surgery may confirm the prediction, or turn the curative data to palliative. On the other hand, evaluation of operability is a global analysis of resectability, performance status and compliance of the patient for surgery. In the initial evaluation, the opinion "non operable" is taken in between 60% and 70% of cases.

Prognosis and classification of oesophageal cancer

In the oesophagus, squamous cell cancer is still the most common type. Adenocarcinoma is located in the lower third of the oesophagus, and for thirty years, rates have been rising rapidly in America and Europe, where it accounts for 30 to 40% of cases [1]. This changing incidence concerns adenocarcinoma in the columnar lined oesophagus, or at the cardia; actually, there is no clear cut difference between these tumours. The overall prognosis of oesophageal cancer is very poor for both tumours, and cure remains unusual: the crude 5 year survival rate is under 10%. The median time of survival, a more relevant clinical estimation of the prognosis, is estimated only in months: the range is between 3 and 12 months for palliative procedures, 12 and 30 months for the so-called curative surgery, 30 and 50 months for the small group of superficial tumours. The curative benefit of surgery concerns only the small group of superficial T1 tumours as illustrated in Japanese series [2]. Superficial cancer represents only 15% and intramucosal (or early) cancer 5% of cases, so that most tumours (T2 to T4) are staged as advanced.

In the management of advanced inoperable oesophageal cancer the objective is a complete relief of the most dramatic symptom – i.e. dysphagia – with minimal morbidity and maximal quality of life. Treatment decision will take into account the degree of dysphagia, graded according to a scoring system, and the performance status, based upon the Karnofsky or WHO scale. The evaluation of the quality of life (QOL) after treatment [3] should be made with adequate methodology. In a recent review of the literature of more than 7,000 references, only 0,6% concerned QOL. Survival following oesophagectomy for oesophageal cancer, extensively reviewed, may be used in reference: the 5 year survival rate is around 20 to 25% [4]. Results have been compared for surgery and non surgical approaches such as radiation, endoscopic procedures or no treatment. In a study conducted in England based on the Nottingham population registry, the respective values of the median survival time for surgery, radiation and intubation were 293, 190 and 100 days; the global 2 year survival rates being 8% [5]. Recent trends in palliation concern the improved efficacy of endoscopic treatment of dysphagia, and the multimodal protocols with concurrent radiation and chemotherapy.

Endoscopic procedures in the palliation of dysphagia

Two major types of endoscopic procedures achieving palliation of dysphagia are luminal debulking through tumour destruction or intubation of the stenosed lumen. Dilatation is a common component in both types. Gastrostomy is an alternative in case of failure of endoscopic palliation of dysphagia.

Luminal dilatation is performed either with bougies (Savary-Gilliard model) or with hydrostatic balloons. The balloon could be preferred on the ground of the selective radial expansion force; however due to its cost (disposable material), bougies are routinely used. Dilatation is performed with the help of a guide wire: angiographic semi flexible guide wires are less traumatic and more "clever" than the metal guide wires. If the stricture is straight, dilatation may be performed without fluoroscopy; in all other situations fluoroscopic control is required. During the first 3 months following radiotherapy, extreme caution in dilatation is required; a diameter of 13 mm should not be exceeded.

Stenting [6, 7], the elective treatment of oesophago-respiratory fistulae, is also an alternative to luminal debulking of tumours in the middle or lower third of the oesophagus, or at the cardia. Conventional stents, made of a reinforced plastic material and allowing a 9 to 12 mm channel are being replaced by metal expandable stents. Their structure is either a mesh, a Z grid, or a coil spring with progressive increase in radial expansion force. They are made of stainless steel, tantalum or various alloys such as nickel and titanium. Expansion after placing the compressed stent is usually ensured by a pull-through catheter. Metal stents have a large lumen (14-20 mm); their placement under fluoroscopy is easy, needing little sedation; a preliminary dilatation is required for tight stenoses. In patients previously treated with radiation and chemotherapy, chronic severe thoracic pain often occurs impairing the quality of life. Furthermore, late complications such as perforation or bleeding may occur. Patients must therefore be selected with care. The drawbacks of metal stents are the high cost and the progressive reduction of lumen patency by tumour invasion and/or inflammation after 2 months. Expandable stents have been coated on one or both sides with silicone, polyethylene, or polyurethane film, covering respiratory fistulae, preventing tumour regrowth, but with an increased risk of dislocation. Metal stents were compared to plastic prostheses in a randomized study; complications were significantly less common in the metal stent group. The coated and uncoated stents may have distinct indications. Squamous cell cancer in the middle oesophagus should be treated with a coated metal stent, preventing tumour in-growth as well as the occurrence of a bronchial fistula. Adenocarcinoma in the distal third should be treated with an uncoated mesh stent, preventing dislocation and sliding in the stomach.

Various procedures have been proposed for intraluminal debulking: snare resection helps in debulking large polypoid tumours, electrocoagulation with the Bicap bipolar probe combines to electrocoagulation and dilatation but the risk of perforation is higher. Brachytherapy, that is intracavitary radiation, is performed with an Iridium 192 or Caesium 137 wire, delivering usually 21 Gy in three sessions at one week intervals. Chemical necrolysis of a polypoid tumour is done at low cost, in the absence of a laser source, with needle catheters and a few ml of absolute ethanol [8]. The Nd: YAG laser photodestruction is actually the best procedure for lumen debulking in polypoid and non circumferential tumours [9]. The morbidity and mortality are lower after laser sessions than after stenting. Laser photoablation must be done in a retrograde rather than an antegrade technique; preliminary dilatation is often required. The risk of perforation is in relation to dilatation, rather than to the laser therapy. The morbidity and mortality are lower with laser sessions, than with stents. Oesophageal perforation occurs in around 1%, usually at the initial dilatation; if it involves the trachea or the bronchial tree, a stent should be urgently placed (plain plastic, or metal coated stent). When the perforation is mediastinal, a naso-gastric tube should be placed immediately; progressive healing occurs usually with parenteral nutrition and antibiotics. Pleural effusion and pneumothorax need immediate drainage and aspiration. Non-thermal laser photodynamic therapy has been suggested for palliation of oesophageal cancer in trials usually conducted with the Photofrin derivative; however the safety efficacy ratio is less favourable [10, 11].

Radiotherapy and chemotherapy

Squamous cell oesophageal cancers have a high rate (70-80%) of tumour response (and corresponding relief of dysphagia) to radiation alone. However the response is often incomplete and the recurrence rate is also very high. Radiation in association with endoscopic treatment (Nd: YAG laser or stent) increases survival as compared to endoscopic treatment in monotherapy [12].

The current focus is on the concurrent administration of chemotherapy. A sound demonstration of the synergy between chemotherapy and radiation has been shown in randomized trials [13]: the survival was significantly longer in the chemoradiation group, as compared to radiation alone. The radiation-chemotherapy multimodal protocol has been first proposed as neo adjuvant, prior to oesophagectomy. Among double or triple drug associations, the 5-FU – cisplatin regimen produced the best safety / efficacy ratio. In neo-adjuvant protocols chemoradiation ensures a complete tumour response in 25-40% of cases as assessed in the operative specimen [14]. However, side effects are common and the increased morbidity and mortality must be taken into account in treatment decision. While concurrent radiation plus chemotherapy proves effective in the treatment of oesophageal squamous cell cancer, the benefit from surgery after the neo-adjuvant treatment is not yet demonstrated in randomized studies. There is nowadays a tendency to select, either the surgical option alone, or the non surgical multimodal protocol.

On the other hand, in adenocarcinoma (oesophagus and cardia) a recent randomized trial [15] comparing surgery alone with a combined preoperative chemotherapy and radiation protocol showed a benefit of the multimodal protocol, the respective values for 3 year survival rate being 32% and 6%, respectively.

Concurrent radiation and chemotherapy was then proposed as an alternative to oesophagectomy in the primary management of squamous cell cancer [16, 17]. The optimal protocol 60 Gy radiation and up to 6 courses of 5-FU – cisplatin. The protocol is also effective in patients with adenocarcinoma. Other treatment modalities have been proposed to act synergistically with concurrent radiation and chemotherapy such as brachytherapy or a laser session after the first chemotherapy course.

Treatment decision in inoperable cancer

In the small group of patients with small stage I tumours (10 to 15%), the curative objective of the treatment is often confirmed by the results. Such cases may be treated by one of the three major endoscopic procedures: Nd: YAG laser photodestruction for polypoid tumours, or strip biopsy [18] for well delineated and small flat neoplastic areas, or photodynamic therapy for flat and large neoplastic poorly delineated areas [19]. There is no sound argument for an adjuvant protocol with chemotherapy and/or radiation in stage I tumours.

Approximately 60 to 70% of patients with oesophageal cancer are not operated on and most of them have advanced cancer. Most tumours in the advanced non operable cancer group are classified as stage III (T3, N+) or IV (M+). Some are classified as stage II a (T2 or T3, N0) or II b (T1, or T2, N+); however, the accuracy of preoperative classification for lymph node invasion is low in spite of echoendoscopy. Therefore for all patients with stage II, III and IV tumours the management calls for palliation, and endoscopic procedures play a major role.

In palliation of dysphagia the two major procedures, stenting and tumour debulking, are complementary. Elements in favour of stenting are: the circular and infiltrative morphology of the tumour; the presence of a oesophago-bronchial fistula; or the development of stenotic fibrosis after repeated laser sessions. Elements in favour of laser photo ablation are: non circular and polypoid pattern of the tumour; the need for lumen debulking before stent positioning; or tumour overgrowth at the proximal or distal end of a stent. Endoscopic procedures are used alone only if there is contra-indication to either radiation or chemotherapy. Indeed in non randomized studies, the non surgical multimodal protocol resulted in survival rates close to those observed in surgical series. Therefore inoperable patients with a satisfactory performance status (Karnofsky score above 50) should enter the concurrent chemotherapy – radiation protocol. Endoscopic dilatation, laser photo ablation, stenting play a role only for specific indications. Laser is used at the initial phase of the treatment only if the tumour is polypoid. Stenting is avoided at the early stage and used later if the tumour response is inadequate. In T4 tumours with a confirmed extension into the bronchial tree, chemotherapy alone is used first; radiation is given later, if there is a marked response of the bronchial wall. In stage IV tumours with distant metastases and mild dysphagia, the treatment is restricted to chemotherapy only.

References

1. Reed PI, Johnston PJ. The changing incidence of oesophageal cancer. *Endoscopy* 1993; 25: 606-8.
2. Nabeya K, Hanaoka T, Li S, Nyumura T. What is the ideal treatment for early oesophageal cancer. *Endoscopy* 1993; 25: 670-1.
3. Gelfand GA, Finlay RJ. Quality of life with carcinoma of the oesophagus. *World J Surg* 1994; 18: 399-405.
4. Bremner RM, DeMeester TR. Surgical treatment of oesophageal carcinoma. *Gastroenterol Clin North Am* 1991; 20: 743-63.
5. Oliver SE, Robertson CS, Logan RF. Oesophageal cancer: a population-based study of survival after treatment. *Br J Surg* 1992; 79: 1321-5.

6. Knyrim K, Wagner J, Bethge N, Keymling M, Vakil N. A controlled trial of an expansible metal stent for palliation of oesophageal obstruction due to inoperable cancer. *N Engl J Med* 1993; 329: 1302-7.
7. Kozarek RA, Ball TJ, Patterson DJ. Metallic self-expanding stent application in the upper gastrointestinal tract: caveats and concerns. *Gastrointest Endosc* 1992; 38: 1-6.
8. Payne James JJ, Spiller RC, Misiewicz JJ, Silk DB. Use of ethanol-induced tumour necrosis to palliate dysphagia in patients with oesophagogastric cancer. *Gastrointestinal Endosc* 1990; 36: 43-6.
9. Lambert R. Cancer in the oesophagus: principles of laser treatment. In: Jensen DM, Brunetaud JM, eds. *Medical laser endoscopy*, Dordrecht: Kluwer 1990: 163-76.
10. Marcon NE. Photodynamic therapy and cancer of the oesophagus. *Semin Oncol* 1994; 21: 20-3.
11. Heier SK, Rothman K, Heier LM, Rosenthal WS. Final results of a randomized trial: photodynamic therapy vs Nd: YAG laser therapy. *Gastroenterology* 1993; 106: A408.
12. Bown SG. Palliation of malignant dysphagia: surgery, radiotherapy, laser, intubation, alone or in combination. *Gut* 1991; 32: 841-4.
13. Herskovic A, Martz K, Al Sarraf L, Leichman L, *et al*. Combined chemotherapy and radiotherapy compared with radiotherapy alone in patients with cancer of the oesophagus. *N Engl J Med* 1992; 1593-8.
14. Forastiere AA, Orringer MB, Perez-Tamayo C, Urba SG, Zahurak M. Preoperative chemoradiation followed by transhiatal oesophagectomy for carcinoma of the oesophagus: final report. *J Clin Oncol* 1993; 11: 1118-23.
15. Walsh TN, Noonan N, Hollywood D, Kelly A, Keeling N, Hennessy TPJ. A comparison of the multimodal therapy and surgery for oesophageal adenocarcinoma. *N Engl J Med* 1996; 335: 462-7.
16. Lambert R. Palliation of carcinoma of the oesophagus. Is there a hope for cure? *Am J Gastroenterol* 1994; 89: S24-S40.
17. Sibille A, Lambert R, Lapeyre B, Souquet JC, Descos F, Ponchon T. Survival following non surgical multimodal treatment for oesophageal squamous cell carcinoma. *Eur J Gastroenterol Hepatol* 1994; 6: 287-92.
18. Inoue H, Endo M, Takeshita K, Kawano T, Goseki N, Takiguchi T. Endoscopic resection of early stage oesophageal cancer. *Surg Endosc* 1991; 5: 59-62.
19. Sibille A, Lambert R, Souquet JC, Sabben G, Descos F. Long term survival after photodynamic therapy for oesophageal cancer. *Gastroenterology* 1995; 108: 337-44.

Treatment of intractable reflux

J. Janssens

University Hospital Leuven, Leuven, Belgium

Summary

Treatment of intractable reflux is strictly speaking a "contradiction in terms". For the clinician, however, the term refers to a clinical situation where the treatment of reflux becomes a real therapeutic challenge in the patient with very severe reflux symptoms (with or without oesophagitis lesions), in the presence of severe oesophagitis (sometimes without manifest reflux symptoms), or in the case of long-lasting recurrent disease. A clear understanding of the various pathogenic factors involved in reflux disease and how they lead to severe symptoms and/or lesions, is essential for an optimal therapeutic approach to the patient with so-called intractable reflux.

Treatment of intractable reflux is strictly speaking a "contradiction in terms". For the clinician, however, the term refers to a clinical situation where the treatment of reflux becomes a real therapeutic challenge in the patient with very severe reflux symptoms (with or without oesophagitis lesions), in the presence of severe oesophagitis (sometimes without manifest reflux symptoms), or in the case of long-lasting recurrent disease.

A clear understanding of the various pathogenic factors involved in reflux disease and how they lead to severe symptoms and/or lesions, is essential for an optimal therapeutic approach to the patient with so-called intractable reflux [1].

Pathogenic factors determining the severity of reflux

Occurrence of reflux

Every reflux episode occurs as a consequence of an incompetent anti-reflux barrier at the gastro-oesophageal junction. The barrier comprises two components: the lower oesophageal sphincter (LOS) and a number of anatomical factors such as the mucosal folds, the angle of His and the intraabdominal position of part of the LOS.

The sphincteric function of the smooth muscle LOS is reinforced by the pinch-cock action of the diaphragmatic crura, which contract and compress the lower oesophagus during increased intraabdominal pressure [2, 3].

Dodds *et al.* have clearly shown that in normal subjects, as well as in patients with pathological reflux, almost all reflux episodes occur as a consequence of one of the three following mechanisms: spontaneous transient lower oesophageal sphincter relaxation (TLOSR), a transient increase in intraabdominal pressure, or a permanent low resting LOS pressure [4].

Patients with reflux disease have an increased number of TLOSR's than normal subjects [5], although some studies (including our own) have found an equal number between normals and patients. More importantly patients with reflux disease have an increased percentage of TLOSR's which are accompanied by reflux, than controls [6, 7]. The reason for this remains unknown. Some studies have suggested a different reaction to the entrance of reflux of the tubular oesophagus which seems to contract in normals, but relaxes in patients with reflux disease, possibly as a consequence of a deficient excitatory cholinergic control [8].

The mechanism underlying the induction of TLOSR's remains incompletely understood. Gastric distension may activate mechanoreceptors located in the subcardial region and induce TLOSR's *via* a vago-vagal reflex. Recent studies [9-11] have suggested that cholecystokinin (CCK) may be one of the neurotransmitters involved in the reflex, as the number of postprandial TLOSR's is increased by exogenous CCK and decreased by CCK-A antagonists such as devazepide and loxiglumide *(figure 1)*. However, there is no existing evidence that abnormal sensitization of the reflex pathway (for example by *Helicobacter pylori* infection) is present in patients with reflux disease.

It has always been accepted that the basal resting pressure of the LOS is an important factor in the prevention of reflux. Indeed, patients with severe oesophagitis have a lower resting pressure than patients with mild oesophagitis or with reflux symptoms only [12]. The overlap, however, between the different groups is so extensive that only in the extreme case of a resting LOS pressure of less than 6 mmHg severe reflux (and oesophagitis) will be present with certainty. When LOS is absent, *i.e.* after proximal partial gastrectomy, reflux is always a severe problem.

The prevalence of a hiatal hernia is known to be high in patients with reflux disease suggesting that the presence of the hernia is permissive for the occurrence of reflux. One factor may be the lack of sphincteric function of the diaphragmatic crura because of the

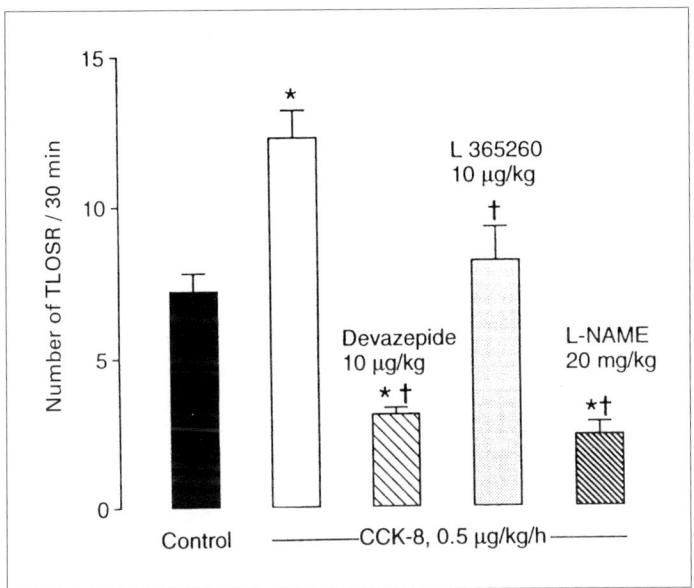

Figure 1. Blockade by devazepide, L365260, and L-NAME of the increase in TLOSR frequency, induced by CCK-8 infusion during gastric distension at 1.56 kPa. *P < 0.05 vs control; †P < 0.05 vs CCK-8 infused alone. (From Boulant et al. [9].)

intrathoracic position of the lower oesophagus. Another probably more important factor is the continuous presence of acid in the hernial sac in close proximity to the sphincter and which enters the oesophagus during the next swallow-induced sphincter relaxation. As shown by Mittal et al. [13], the phenomenon clearly interferes with an efficient acid clearance.

Clearance of refluxate

The clearance of the refluxed material from the oesophageal lumen is a two step phenomenon: volume clearance by gravity and by oesophageal peristalsis, and chemical clearance by bicarbonate in the swallowed saliva. In case of a reflux event almost all acid material is already cleared from the oesophagus after the first peristaltic contraction; but the remaining acid that sticks to the wall as a thin layer requires chemical neutralisation by alkaline saliva [14, 15]. Without an efficient initial volume clearance the small amount of bicarbonate in saliva will not be able to neutralise the remaining acid in the oesophagus.

Volume clearance is mainly due to primary swallow-induced peristaltic contractions. However, secondary peristalsis induced by the presence of a refluxed bolus seems to be also very important for efficient clearance, especially at night. A minimal amplitude of 30 mm Hg in the distal oesophagus is required for clearance by peristalsis, but the peristaltic nature of the contraction is even more important. Patients with gastro-oesophageal reflux disease have an increased rate of failure of primary peristalsis and this increases with the severity of the reflux disease [16]. There is also a concomitant decrease in mean peristaltic amplitude and this decrease is more pronounced in case of severe oesophagitis

[17]. Schoeman *et al.* have shown that secondary peristalsis is almost equally important as primary peristalsis for oesophageal clearance [18]. These authors also showed that the threshold for induction of secondary peristalsis is higher in reflux patients than in controls, and that these secondary contractions more frequently have an abnormal peristaltic progression in the patients [19] *(figure 2)*.

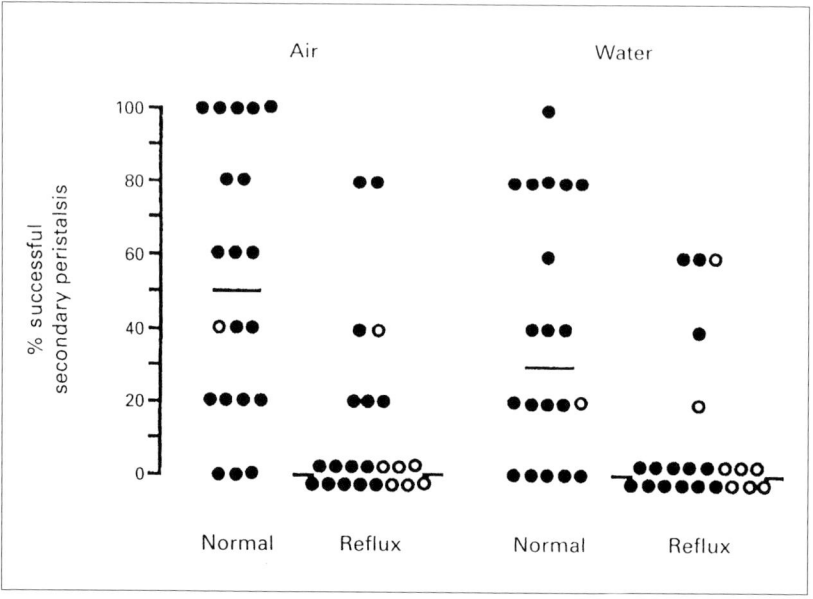

Figure 2. Percentage of secondary peristalsis with air and water bolus injections. Each point represents the proportion of normal secondary peristaltic responses (out of five tests) for each subject. Subjects with normal primary peristalsis are represented by the filled circles and those with abnormal primary peristalsis with the open circles. The horizontal bars show median values. The frequency of the responses for both stimuli was significantly less in the reflux patients than in normal volunteers (p ≤ 0.003). (From Schoeman and Holloway [18].)

Irritation potential of the refluxate

Numerous studies have shown that acid and pepsin are the most important noxious factors in the refluxate and are mainly responsible for the symptoms and lesions. The effect of acid concentration on the induction of reflux symptoms was studied by Smith *et al.* by means of acid perfusion of various pH's and for various durations in the oesophagus of patients with reflux symptoms and a positive Bernstein test [20].

The lower the pH, the more likely it is for reflux symptoms to occur, and the dose-response curve seemed to plateau at pH values above 4. The lower the pH of the perfusate, the more rapidly symptoms occurred.

If one tries, however, to correlate the appearance of reflux symptoms with the occurrence of reflux episodes on a 24 h pH monitoring, the issue becomes confused. While most symptom episodes (but not all) correlate in time with a reflux episode on the recording, many more apparently similar reflux episodes are present which do not induce symptoms. We have studied this problem by determining the total acid burden (pH x time) during a given time period preceding symptomatic reflux episodes as compared to the acid burden preceding asymptomatic reflux episodes: we have found a significantly higher acid burden in the 20 minute – period that preceded symptomatic reflux episodes compared to asymptomatic reflux events [21]. Therefore the total amount of acid contact during a given time period is an important factor in the production of reflux symptoms, in the same way as it is important for the production of oesophagitis lesions (but the latter phenomenon was already known previously).

The noxious effect of acid (and pepsin) on oesophageal mucosa has been studied in many *in vitro* and *in vivo* experiments in several animal species including cat, dog, rabbit and opossum [22]. Functional changes in oesophageal mucosal integrity occur very early in the process of acid perfusion, before any significant histological damage can be detected by conventional techniques. The relation between amount of acid and lesions has also been demonstrated in humans as there is a clear correlation between the acid load in the oesophagus (expressed as percent time of pH below 4 during 24 h pH monitoring) and the degree of oesophagitis [23]. Both day time and night time (supine) reflux is noxious to the oesophageal mucosa; night time reflux is supposed to be the more harmful as salivary secretion and oesophageal motility are reduced at night, mainly due to absence of swallowing [24]. Severe oesophagitis and Barrett's are mainly found in patients with very prolonged upright and supine exposure; and conversely there exists a linear correlation between healing rate of oesophagitis lesions and the degree of acid inhibition by antisecretory drugs, the higher this acid inhibition, the better the healing rate [25].

There is no evidence to suppose that gastric acid output is higher in patients with reflux disease as compared to normal controls, and there is no relationship between severity of the oesophagitis and gastric acid output [26]. It does not mean, however, that patients with Zollinger-Ellison syndrome may not have very severe oesophagitis [27]. Patients with delayed gastric emptying also seem to have an increased acid exposure to the oesophageal mucosa; and delayed gastric emptying was reported to be associated with reduced responsiveness to medical therapy and with failure after anti-reflux surgery [28].

The noxious effect of so-called alkaline reflux, in particular the noxious effect of bile acids on oesophageal mucosa is controversial. Theoretically bile salts may or may not be harmful to the oesophageal mucosa depending on the pH: at low pH the harmful effect of hydrochloric acid can be aggravated by conjugated bile acids; while unconjugated bile acids (and trypsin), which are not harmful at low pH, could be noxious at neutral pH [29]. In a study by Gotley *et al.* in patients with pathological reflux, continuous aspiration of oesophageal content showed that concentrations of bile acids sufficiently high to be deleterious to the mucosa are present in only a small minority of patients [30]. In a more recent study by Champion *et al.*, however, the Bilitec® system was used to monitor concentrations of bilirubin in the refluxate; the study clearly showed an increased exposure of bilirubin to the oesophageal mucosa in patients with reflux disease as compared to normals, the exposure being particularly high in patients with Barrett's mucosa *(figure 3)*. As there was no significant difference in the percent time that the intraoesophageal pH was above 7 between reflux patients and normals, the authors concluded that the term "alkaline reflux" was a misnomer and should be abandoned [31].

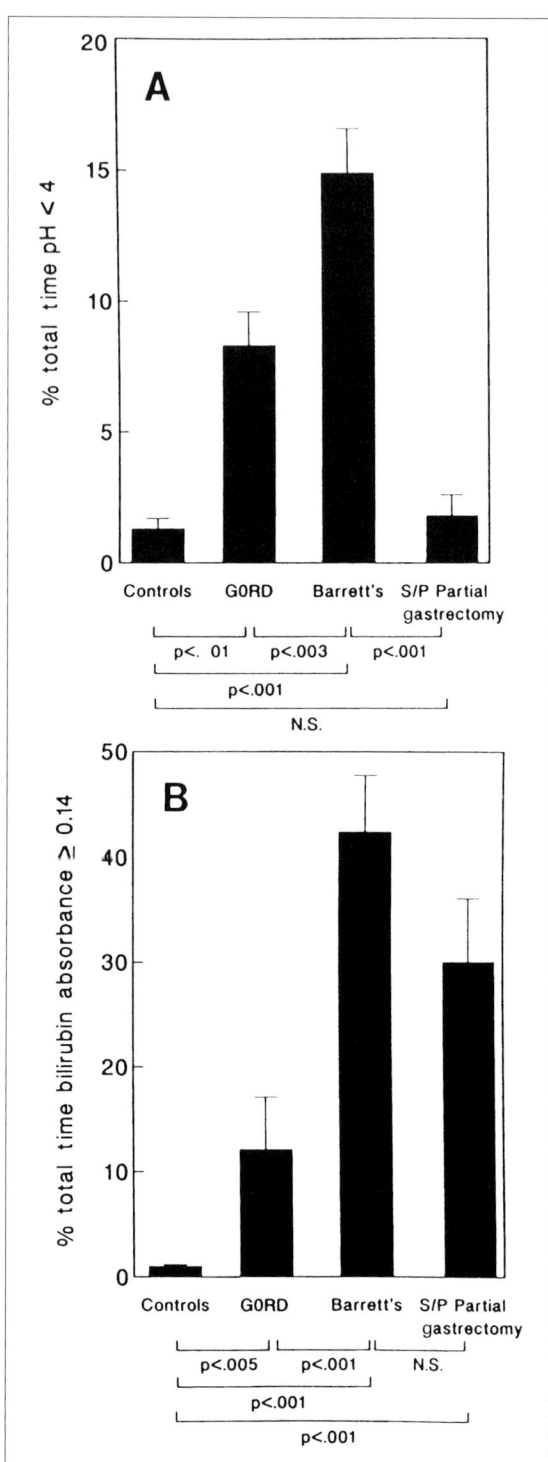

Figure 3. Group means ± SE for (A) acid reflux (percent of total time pH was < 4) and (B) DGOR (percent of time bilirubin absorbance was ≥ 0.14) for the four study populations. Both acid reflux and DGOR increased significantly with the severity of GORD with both values, being greatest in patients with Barrett's oesophagus. As expected, post-partial gastrectomy patients had small amounts of acid reflux, similar to healthy controls. On the other hand, the amount of DGOR nearly approached the values found in patients with Barrett's oesophagus. (From Champion et al. [31].)

Oesophageal mucosal defence mechanisms

Saliva contains a number of substances such as mucin, growth factors and prostaglandins, which are known to have a mucosal protective effect. A layer of mucus from saliva and oesophageal submucosal glands forms a defence layer by preventing diffusion of larger molecules such as pepsin (but not hydrochloric acid), to the epithelial cells. Although part of the diffused acid is neutralised by bicarbonate in the mucus, the major barrier to acid diffusion is formed by the superficial cell layers of the oesophageal mucosa. A recently defined glycoconjugate material, probably synthesised in the mucosal cells and stored in intracellular membrane-bound vesicles before being secreted into the intercellular spaces, is probably more important for the mucosal barrier function than the tight junctions between cells [32]. Several homeostatic mechanisms that regulate intracellular pH, an adequate blood supply and the regeneration capacity of the mucosa are all important factors in the mucosal defence.

It is unknown to what extent an intrinsic defect of the mucosal defence contributes to the severity of oesophageal lesions in patients with reflux disease.

Treatment of intractable disease

Treatment of intractable symptoms

Heartburn and acid regurgitation, when predominant symptoms, are quite specific but not very sensitive for reflux disease. Many other, less specific symptoms including cough, nausea and vomiting, hoarseness, hiccups, angina-like chest pain may also be due to reflux, and some of these symptoms such as angina-like chest pain may be very disabling.

Only one third of patients with typical reflux symptoms will have endoscopic evidence of oesophagitis. More importantly, neither the pattern nor the severity of the symptoms can be used to predict the presence or absence of oesophagitis [33, 34].

There are many arguments in favour of the idea that the total acidity with which the oesophageal mucosa is in contact, is the main determinant in the production of symptoms: reflux symptoms are more readily induced by solutions of low pH; the lower the pH of the solution, the shorter the contact time needed to induce symptoms; the total acid burden to the oesophageal mucosa "primes" the mucosa and makes it more sensitive to the next reflux episode; and the spatio-temporal characteristics, especially the extent of the reflux, are also important for symptom production.

It thus seems logical to accept that the higher the acid suppression by antisecretory agents, the more successful will be the symptom reduction. In selected cases antireflux surgery may be indicated to adequately treat symptoms, even in the absence of endoscopic evidence of oesophagitis.

Symptoms, however, also depend on oesophageal sensitivity to acid and this sensitivity may vary considerably intra- but also interindividually. Galmiche *et al.* have identified a subgroup of reflux patients characterized by a normal acid exposure to the oesophagus, despite a statistically significant relationship between symptoms and reflux episodes detected during 24 h pH monitoring [35, 36] *(figure 4)*. These patients presented with the same symptom pattern as patients with non-erosive reflux disease. While reflux patients usually display a normal or even reduced sensation to mechanical distension, some patients with acid hypersensitivity have a very low threshold for mechanical stimulation, suggesting that they are more sensitive to a variety of stimuli [37].

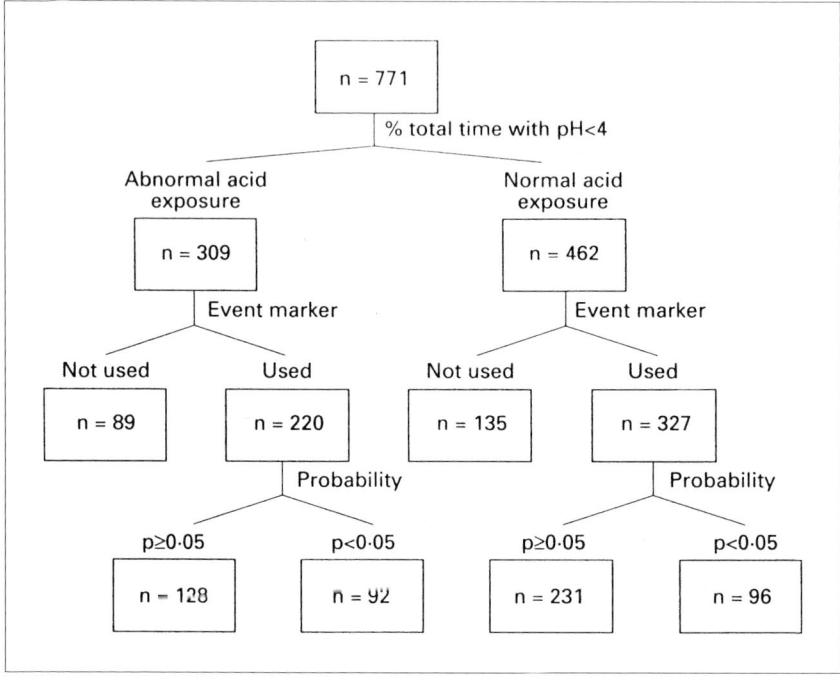

Figure 4. Frequency of patients with normal oesophageal exposure to acid and statistically significant association between symptoms and reflux episodes during 24 hour pH monitoring in a series of 771 consecutive patients referred for 24 hour pH monitoring. Some patients were investigated on several occasions (n = number of patients). (From Shi et al. [36].)

A subgroup of patients with angina-like chest pain of non-cardiac origin due to reflux belong to this group of patients with the irritable oesophagus syndrome [35, 38]. As patients with an acid hypersensitive oesophagus feel acid reflux of acidity and duration well within the limits of physiological reflux, profound acid suppression and even anti-reflux surgery may be needed to control their symptoms.

Treatment of intractable oesophagitis

Numerous data in the literature have shown that greater acid exposure leads to more severe oesophagitis, and that healing rates of erosive oesophagitis correlate with acid suppression over a 24 h period [25]. In case of severe oesophagitis control of daytime and night-time acid secretion is essential for clinical success.

As discussed previously, several conditions are expected to be accompanied by increased oesophageal acid exposure, and thus constitute an increased risk for severe oesophagitis: a very low basal resting pressure of the LOS; the presence of a hiatal hernia; low amplitude and disordered peristaltic progression of oesophageal contractions; delayed gastric emptying; supine reflux and the like. In case of severe oesophagitis, these abnormalities should be looked for and treated accordingly.

An excessive amount of bile acids in the refluxate seems to increase the risk of development of Barrett's epithelium. In contrast to other patients with reflux oesophagitis, patients with Barrett's seem to have a lower sensitivity to acid. This may explain why they remain asymptomatic for a long time despite severe lesions and prolonged acid exposure [39, 40]. The epidemiological finding that 95% of patients with Barrett's oesophagus are never diagnosed also suggests that most of these patients do not develop sufficiently severe symptoms to trigger endoscopy [41]. The lack of severe reflux symptoms in Barrett's patients may have consequences for therapy, as elimination of reflux symptoms in these patients does not guarantee adequate control of acid exposure [42]. Since acid exposure is thought to be one of the major determinants in the development of Barrett's, dysplasia and adenocarcinoma, the endpoint of therapy in these patients should be adequate acid suppression, which can only be objectively measured by 24 h pH monitoring.

Treatment of long-lasting and recurrent disease

Current medical therapy, although highly effective for the treatment of symptoms and/or lesions, has almost no effect on the pathogenic abnormalities that underlie the occurrence of reflux. It is not surprising therefore that despite efficient medical therapy, reflux disease is a chronic disease in most patients, with early recurrence after the end of medical treatment. Only in the early stages of pathological reflux the disease may (spontaneously?) fluctuate, which may explain that long-lasting remissions after short-term initial therapy have been described in about 40% of the patients [43].

In long-lasting and/or recurrent disease the appropriate medical therapy may differ for erosive and for non-erosive reflux disease. As a consequence, early endoscopy is mandatory during the course [44].

If endoscopy shows erosive oesophagitis, proton-pump inhibitors (PPI's) are the most appropriate medical therapy. They are the only effective therapy in cases of severe oesophagitis. In mild oesophagitis PPI's are still the most effective and cost-effective medical treatment [45, 46]. In the latter group, symptom control can be a guide to therapy, as it is highly unusual to find substantial endoscopic oesophagitis if symptoms are adequately relieved [47]. It is still debated whether low-grade oesophagitis can be adequately treated by half dose PPI's, or by PPI's on demand. Antireflux surgery should be considered as an alternative, depending on effectiveness of symptom control by medication, doses needed, costs, and preference of the patient.

In case of long-lasting and/or recurrent symptoms without endoscopic evidence of erosive oesophagitis, the therapeutic strategy is less clear. As the risk of developing significant oesophagitis lesions is minimal in these patients, treatment of symptoms at lowest cost seems appropriate. The step-up mode of therapy starting with life-style modifications and adding subsequently H$_2$-receptor antagonists or prokinetics and PPI's is still widely accepted [48].

However, the socio-economics of these various treatments, including surgery, have not been studied thus far.

References

1. Galmiche JP, Janssens J. The pathophysiology of gastro-oesophageal reflux disease: an overview. *Scand J Gastroenterol* 1995; 30 (suppl 211): 7-18.
2. Mittal RK, Rochester DF, McCallum RW. Electrical and mechanical activity in the human lower oesophageal sphincter during diaphragmatic contraction. *J Clin Invest* 1988; 81: 1182-9.
3. Mittal RK, Rochester DF, McCallum RW. Sphincteric action of the diaphragm during a relaxed lower oesophageal sphincter in humans. *Am J Physiol* 1989; 256: G139-G144.
4. Dodds WJ, Dent J, Hogan WJ, et al. Mechanism of gastro-oesophageal reflux in patients with reflux oesophagitis. *N Engl J Med* 1982; 307: 1547-52.
5. Aktaridis G, Snape W, Cohen S. Lower oesophageal sphincter pressure as an index of gastro-oesophageal acid reflux. *Dig Dis Sci* 1981; 26: 993-8.
6. Mittal RK, McCallum RW. Characteristics and frequency of transient relaxations of the lower oesophageal sphincter in patients with reflux oesophagitis. *Gastroenterology* 1988; 95: 593.
7. Freidin N, Fisher MJ, Taylor W, et al. Sleep and nocturnal acid reflux in normal subjects and patients with reflux oesophagitis. *Gut* 1991; 32: 1275-9.
8. Janssens J, Sifrim D. New insights in the pathophysiology of primary motility disorders of the oesophagus. *Verhandelingen Kon Acad Geneesk België* 1997; 59: 208-26.
9. Boulant J, Fioramonti J, Dapoigny M, Bommelaer G, Bueno L. Cholecystokinin and nitric oxide in transient lower oesophageal sphincter relaxation to gastric distension in dogs. *Gastroenterology* 1994; 107: 1059-66.
10. Zerbib F, Bruley des Varannes S, D'Amato M, Scarpignato C, Galmiche JP. Effect of the CCK-A receptor antagonist loxiglumide on gastric tone and transient lower oesophageal sphincter relaxations in humans. *Gastroenterology* 1997; 112: A857.
11. Boulant J, Mathieu S, D'Amato M, Abergel A, Dapoigny M, Bommelaer G. Cholecystokinin in transient lower oesophageal relaxations due to gastric distension in man. *Gut* 1997; 40: 575-81.
12. Kahrilas PJ, Dodds WJ, Hogan WJ, et al. Oesophageal peristaltic dysfunction in peptic oesophagitis. *Gastroenterology* 1986; 91: 897-904.
13. Mittal RK, Lange RC, McCallum RW. Identification and mechanism of delayed oesophageal acid clearance in subjects with hiatus hernia. *Gastroenterology* 1987; 92: 130-5.
14. Helm JF, Dodds WJ, Pele LR, et al. Effect of oesophageal emptying and saliva on clearance of acid from the oesophagus. *N Engl J Med* 1984; 310: 284-8.
15. Helm JF, Dodds WJ, Hogan WJ, et al. Acid neutralizing capacity of human saliva. *Gastroenterology* 1982; 83: 69-74.
16. Kahrilas PJ, Dodds WJ, Hogan WJ. Effect of peristaltic dysfunction on oesophageal volume clearance. *Gastroenterology* 1988; 94: 73-80.
17. Kahrilas PJ. Oesophageal motor activity and acid clearance. *Gastroenterol Clin North Am* 1990; 19: 537-50.
18. Schoeman MN, Tipett MD, Akkermans LMA, Dent J, Holloway RH. Mechanisms of gastro-oesophageal reflux in ambulant healthy human subjects. *Gastroenterology* 1995; 108: 83-91.
19. Schoeman MN, Holloway RH. Integrity and characteristics of secondary oesophageal peristalsis in patients with gastro-oesophageal reflux disease. *Gut* 1995; 36: 499-504.

20. Smith JL, Opekum AR, Larkai R, Graham DY. Sensitivity of the oesophageal mucosa to pH in gastro-oesophageal reflux disease. *Gastroenterology* 1989; 96: 683-9.
21. Janssens J, Vantrappen G, Vos R, Ghillebert G. The acid burden over an extended period preceding a reflux episode is a major determinant in the development of heartburn. *Gastroenterology* 1992; 102: A90.
22. Ferguson DJ, Sanchez-Palomera E, Sako Y, Clatworthy HW, Toon RW, Wangensteen OH. Studies on experimental oesophagitis. *Surgery* 1950; 28: 1022-39.
23. Hixson LJ, Kelley CL, Jones WN, Tuohy CD. Current trends in the pharmacotherapy for gastro-oesophageal reflux disease. *Arch Intern Med* 1992; 152: 717-23.
24. Orr WC, Johnson LF, Robinson MG. Effect of sleep on swallowing, oesophageal peristaltism and acid clearance. *Gastroenterology* 1984; 86: 814-9.
25. Bell NJ, Burget D, Howden CW, Wilkinson J, Hunt RH. Appropriate acid suppression for the management of gastro-oesophageal reflux disease. *Digestion* 1992; 51 (suppl 1): 59-67.
26. Hirschowitz BI. A critical analysis with appropriate controls of gastric acid and pepsin secretion in clinical oesophagitis. *Gastroenterology* 1991; 101: 1149-58.
27. Miller LS, Vinayek R, Frucht H, Gardner JD, Jensen RT, Maton PN. Reflux oesophagitis in patients with Zollinger-Ellison syndrome. *Gastroenterology* 1990; 98: 341-6.
28. Scarpignato C, Franze A. Oesophageal exposure to acid in GERD patients with and without delayed gastric emptying. Effect of cisapride. *Hepato-Gastroenterol* 1992; 39: 91-2.
29. Vaezi MF, Singh S, Richter JE. Role of acid and duodenogastric reflux in oesophageal mucosal injury: a review of animal and human studies. *Gastroenterology* 1995; 108: 1897-907.
30. Gotley DC, Morgan AP, Ball D, Owen RW, Cooper MJ. Composition of gastro-oesophageal refluxate. *Gut* 1991; 32: 1093-9.
31. Champion G, Richter JE, Vaezi MF, Singh S, Alexander R. Duodenogastro-oesophageal reflux: relationship to pH and importance in Barrett's oesophagus. *Gastroenterology* 1994; 107: 747-54.
32. Orlando RC, Lacy ER, Tobey NA, Cowart K. Barriers to paracellular permeability in rabbit oesophageal epithelium. *Gastroenterology* 1992; 102: 910-23.
33. Palmer ED. The hiatus hernia-oesophagitis-oesophageal stricture complex. Twenty-year prospective study. *Am J Med* 1968; 44: 566-79.
34. Winters C Jr, Spurling TJ, Chobanian SJ, et al. Barrett's oesophagus. A prevalent, occult complication of gastro-oesophageal reflux disease. *Gastroenterology* 1987; 92: 118-24.
35. Galmiche JP, Scarpignato C. Oesophageal sensitivity to acid in patients with non-cardiac chest pain: is the oesophagus hypersensitive? *Eur J Gastroenterol Hepatol* 1995; 7: 1152-9.
36. Shi G, Bruley des Varannes S, Scarpignato C, Le Rhun M, Galmiche JP. Reflux-related symptoms in patients with normal oesophageal exposure to acid. *Gut* 1995; 37: 457-64.
37. Vantrappen G, Janssens J, Ghillebert G. The irritable oesophagus – a frequent cause of angina-like pain. *Lancet* 1987; I: 1232-4.
38. Janssens J, Vantrappen G. Irritable oesophagus. *Am J Med* 1992; 92 (suppl 5A): 27S-32S.
39. Johnson DA, Winters C, Spurling TJ, et al. Oesophageal acid sensitivity in Barrett's oesophagus. *J Clin Gastroenterol* 1987; 9: 23-7.
40. Murphy PP, Johnston BT, Collins JSA. Mucosal sensitivity and salivary response to infused acid in patients with columnar-lined oesophagus. *Eur J Gastroenterol Hepatol* 1994; 6: 901-5.
41. Cameron AJ, Zinsmeister AR, Ballard DJ, et al. Prevalence of columnar-lined (Barrett's) oesophagus. Comparison of population-based clinical and autopsy findings. *Gastroenterology* 1990; 99: 918-22.
42. Katzka DA, Castell DO. Successful elimination of reflux symptoms does not insure adequate control of acid reflux in patients with Barrett's oesophagus. *Am J Gastroenterol* 1994; 89: 989-91.
43. Lieberman DA. Medical therapy for chronic reflux oesophagitis. *Arch Intern Med* 1987; 147: 1717-20.

44. Hillman AL, Bloom BS, Fendrick AM, Schwartz JS. Cost and quality effects of alternative treatments for persistent gastro-oesophageal reflux disease. *Arch Intern Med* 1992; 152: 1467-72.
45. Green JRB, Bate CM, Copeman MB, Taylor MD. A comparison of the cost-effectiveness of omeprazole and ranitidine in reflux oesophagitis. *Br J Med Econom* 1995; 8: 157-69.
46. Sridhar S, Huang J, O'Brien BJ, Hunt RH. Clinical economics review: cost effectiveness of treatment alternatives for gastro-oesophageal reflux disease. *Aliment Pharmacol Ther* 1996; 10: 865-73.
47. Carlsson R, Galmiche JP, Dent J, Lundell L, Frison L. Prognostic factors influencing relapse of oesophagitis during maintenance therapy with antisecretory drugs: a meta-analysis of long-term omeprazole trials. *Aliment Pharmacol Ther* 1997: in press.
48. Tytgat GNJ, Janssens J, Reynolds JC, Wienbeck M. Update on the pathophysiology and management of gastro-oesophageal reflux disease: the role of prokinetic therapy. *Eur J Gastroenterol Hepatol* 1996; 8: 603-11.

Causes and consequences of intestinal failure: the model of the short bowel

B. Messing

Groupe hospitalier Saint-Lazare, Lariboisière, Fernand Widal, et INSERM U 290, Paris, France

Summary

Intestinal failure is a condition in which the intestine is unable to process sufficient food to maintain adequate nutritional status. Chronic failure results mainly from extensive resection of the small intestine as a consequence of infarction, or Crohn's disease. Definition of intestinal failure following intestinal resection should take into account measurement of the remaining small bowel, the three main types of anastomosis: end-enterostomy (type I), jejuno-colonic (type II) and jejuno-ileocolonic anastomosis (type III), plus an evaluation of the length of the remaining colon. Short bowel which induces chronic intestinal failure leaves a remnant of small bowel of less than 150 cm; less than 50% of the shortest length of a normal adult small bowel. Severe intestinal failure can be expected with a small bowel length of less than 100 cm. Measurement of plasma concentration of citrulline, an amino acid produced in enterocytes, is a promising biomarker of the enterocyte mass because it is highly correlated with the length of the remaining small bowel in the short bowel model. Current management of chronic intestinal failure is parenteral nutrition associated with fluid and food optimisation for maximal absorption, where the colon plays a crucial role. Complementary options to home parenteral nutrition include trophic factors and surgical procedures to enhance function of the remnant to help weaning from parenteral nutrition. An alternative option is intestinal transplantation.

Definition of intestinal failure

Intestinal failure is defined as "the reduction in the functioning gut mass below the minimal amount necessary for the absorption of nutrients" [1]. Oral failure is defined as the reduction in the oral intake below the minimal amount necessary to maintain protein-energy equilibrium taking into account the patient's usual activity [2]. Both situations lead to protein-energy malnutrition, but intestinal failure due to malabsorption of solute results in addition in diarrhoea, fluid and electrolyte losses *(figure 1)*. Intestinal failure is defined as a condition in which there is inadequate absorption of solutes derived from the digested products of the ingested food [3]. A pitfall arises when intestinal failure is associated with oral failure, because the latter can mask the former. Present treatment option of intestinal failure is Home Parenteral Nutrition (HPN) [4]. In the present overview, short bowel, which is the main cause of chronic intestinal failure, is used as a model [5].

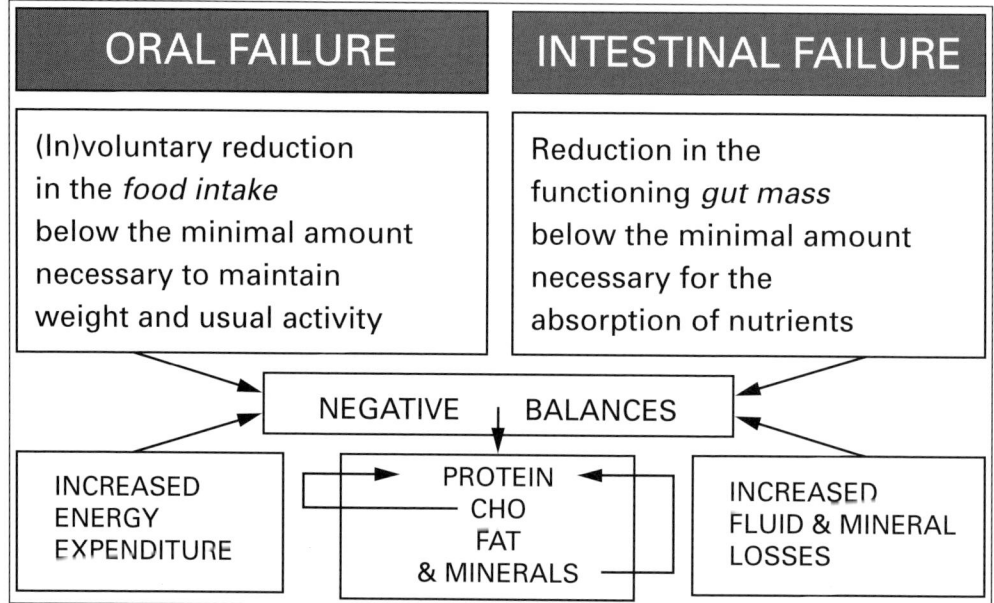

Figure 1. Oral and intestinal failures. Definition and consequences. Oral and intestinal failures can interact, the former can make the latter underexpressed. Both conditions lead to protein-energy malnutrition whereas the latter induces fluid and mineral deficiencies.

Causes of intestinal failure

Severe chronic intestinal failure needing HPN has two major causes: intestinal small bowel motor malfunction, mainly intestinal obstruction, and intestinal malabsorption syndrome *(figure 2)*. Both conditions can be present simultaneously, as in small bowel fistulas which represented 10-20% of HPN indications [1, 5]. Intestinal obstruction may be with or without stenosis. Stenosis is mainly seen with cancer, Crohn's disease or radiation enteritis; obstruction in the absence of stenosis is due to the chronic intestinal pseudo obstruction (CIPO) syndrome. It has a large variety of causes: either primary (mainly seen in childhood: *e.g.*, mitochondrial diseases, myenteric plexus abnormalities) or secondary (mainly seen in adulthood: *e.g.*, scleroderma, paraneoplastic syndrome, complication of

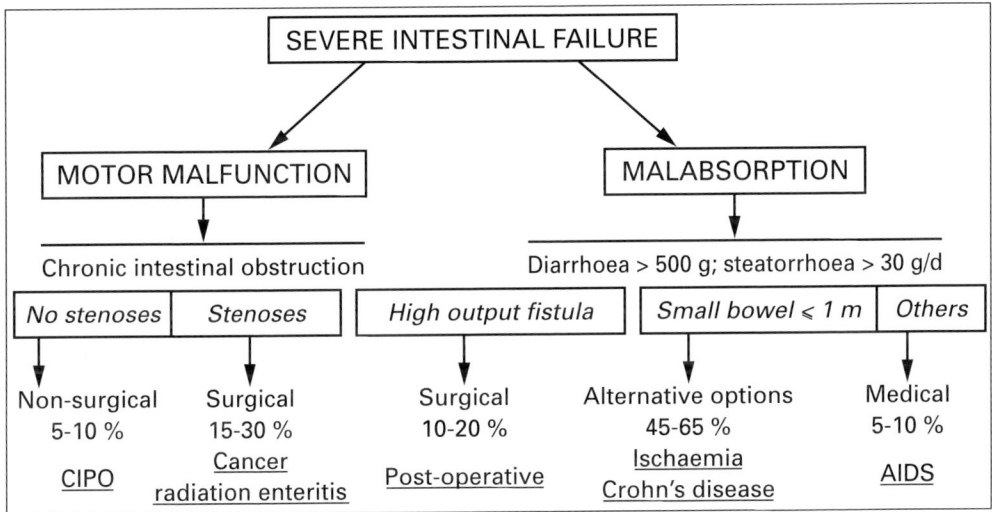

Figure 2. Causes of intestinal failure leading to home parenteral nutrition treatment (HPN). HPN indications in percent, with at the bottom, main diagnosis leading to it. CIPO = chronic intestinal pseudo obstruction.

chemotherapy). Severe malabsorptive intestinal failure is mainly secondary to total or massive small bowel resection. Main causes of short bowel are: (a) severe Crohn's disease or radiation enteritis (50% of cases), (b) mesenteric infarction (30% of cases) due to trauma, volvulus, splanchnic vessel (arterial or venous) occlusion and (c) cancer (20%) [4-7, 9-11]. Short bowel represents 50% of non-cancer, non-AIDS HPN indications [4-7] and more than 75% of long term HPN indications [5]. Non-surgical severe malabsorption syndrome needing HPN also has several causes: *e.g.*, total villous atrophy such as coeliac sprue, AIDS or lymphoma. In the 14 approved adult centres in France, new HPN patients in the years 1993-1995 (n = 524) had been nearly equal incidence of six following diagnosies: Crohn's disease, mesenteric infarction, radiation enteritis, cancer, AIDS and miscellaneous (the latter included post-operative complications, CIPO and severe medical (non-AIDS) malabsorption syndrome [7].

Aetiology, definition and measurement of short bowel

Aetiology

Short bowel occurs in up to 15% of adults undergoing surgical resection [12], the most frequent cause in the United Kingdom being Crohn's disease [10] and in France ischaemia [11]. Necrotizing enterocolitis and congenital intestinal anomalies are the major causes of extensive intestinal resection in children [13, 14]. In adults, the incidence of short bowel requiring long term HPN support is estimated at 2 per 1,000,000 per year [4-6, 9].

Definition

Since the usual length of small bowel ranges in adults from three to eight metres, depending on whether or not it is measured at surgery, autopsy or from X-ray films, short bowel is more appropriately defined by the length of remnant, rather than by the extent of resection [3, 10]. Short bowel can be defined as an extra-duodenal remnant length of less than 150-200 cm, *i.e.* less than half the lower normal small bowel length in adults [10]. To avoid turning "short bowel" into a misnomer, its definition should indicate both the length of the remaining small bowel and the three main short-bowel types of anastomosis, *i.e.* end-enterostomy -type I, jejunocolonic -type II or jejunoileocolonic -type III [15-17]. Indeed, these main short-bowel types of anastomosis indicate not only the site of the small bowel remnant, *i.e.* jejunum *versus* ileum, but also the preservation of either part of colon (type II), or an ileal remnant with ileocaecal valve and colon (type III), which significantly improve oral water-mineral and/or energy balance of absorption [17-19].

Measurement of bowel remnant

Accurate assessment of the amount of intestinal remnant is difficult. In the small bowel an accurate but indirect measurement can be made along the antimesenteric border of the small intestine on a barium meal follow-through with an opisometer, a device used for measuring distances on maps [20]. Opisometry has been shown to correlate significantly with peroperative measurements of small bowel remnant lengths [20]. In the colon, the length of which is very variable, the bowel is arbitrarily divided into seven sections assumed to be of equal length: each part thus represents 14% of the large bowel. The length of a colonic remnant can be then expressed as a percentage of the total [19].

Effects of intestinal resection

Some essential aspects of gastrointestinal physiology will be reviewed to understand the main effects of intestinal resection.

Gastric function

After the first 30 to 60 min following a meal, physiologic and constant rates of gastric emptying are set up at a maximum of 6 ml/min for acaloric fluid and electrolytes and at 3.0 cal/min for caloric loads [21]. Liquids, according to their osmolality, empty more rapidly from the gastric reservoir than solids. Gastric emptying slows down when the chyme enters the ileum and preservation of the colon after major small intestinal resection exerts a braking effect on the rate of *early* gastric emptying of liquid [22]. Gastric emptying is therefore accelerated in end-jejunostomy patients in comparison with patients with a jejunocolonic, or jejuno-ileocolonic type of anastomosis [22]. Following large intestinal resection, there is hypergastrinaemia and gastric acid hypersecretion which contribute to the massive fluid and electrolyte losses and later on to the possible occurrence of peptic ulceration [3, 10].

Small bowel function

Optimal absorption of nutrients requires adequate time of contact with the absorptive sites of the small intestine. Therefore it is worth noting that propulsion is three times slower in the ileum than in the jejunum [23] and that this effect is observed when the distal ileum is retained, even in the absence of the ileocoecal valve [24]. The infusion of fat in the dog jejunum [25] or the human ileum exerted a braking effect on the upper small intestine transit time [26]. Small bowel transit time (head of the column) was faster than in controls for liquid in short bowel patients with and without a colon and for solids in those without a colon [22]. Consistent with a slower gastric emptying for solid proteins in comparison to liquid proteins, we demonstrated in end-jejunostomy patients better jejunal absorption of the former (caseins) in comparison to the latter (lactoglobulins) type of proteins [27].

Approximately 50% of the 18,000 to 20,000 ml of extracellular body water enters and turns over per day in the small bowel. Reabsorption of fluids is nearly complete at the end of the ileum, since only 800 ml per day enters the colon. However, depending on whether a meal has high or a low osmolality, much of the fluid is absorbed in the proximal or distal part of the small intestine, respectively [28]. Water movement follows active transport of ions (mainly sodium) and nutrients (mainly glucose and peptides or amino-acids). Water-sodium movement into the lumen can be dramatically increased through either high osmolality molecules (*e.g.* lactose) [29] or hypo-osmotic water [30] because both induce a water-sodium serosa –> lumen movement which is aimed at (re)establishing an iso-osmotic intraluminal fluid. This movement is greater into the jejunum than in the ileum through leaky intercellular junctions. Net movement of water across the small bowel is therefore the result of two opposite drives: absorption (Na-glucose, Na-peptides) and ionic back diffusion. It has been estimated that the efficiency of water absorption is 44% and 70% of the ingested load in the jejunum and ileum, respectively; for sodium the corresponding estimates are 13% and 72% [3, 31]. Patients who have undergone ileal resection have a reduced capacity to absorb sodium chloride, particularly when there is a concentration gradient between lumen and plasma [32]. Hence the ileum plays a major role in conservation of fluid and electrolytes which can only be partially compensated for by the preservation of the colon in the short bowel syndrome.

Unique functions of the ileum

B12 and bile salts are actively absorbed only in the distal ileum. Bile salt concentration reach their micellar concentration following a (fat) meal only if bile salts are actively absorbed and recycled enterohepatically. Malabsorption of long chain triglycerides (steatorrhoea) and of fat soluble vitamins follows isolated ileal resection of more than 100 cm [33]. Disruption of the enterohepatic cycle allows increased quantities of bile salts to enter the colon which reduces the ability of the colon to absorb salt and water. In addition, colonic flora produces deoxy bile salts, which induce colonic water secretion. Increased diarrhoea follows. By contrast, jejunal resection with preservation of the ileum (usually associated in clinical practice with the preservation of the ileocaecal valve), does not induce either fat malabsorption, or significant diarrhoea.

Adaptive function of the colon

The colon absorbs water and sodium very efficiently up to 95% after a constant caecal infusion of 6,000 ml per day [34, 35]. This rate is probably reduced by the malabsorbed food components which enter the colon after an ileal resection. On the contrary, non absorbed carbohydrates can be fermented into short chain fatty acids (SCFAs) through colonic bacterial metabolism; SCFAs absorption follows, a process which increases water, sodium and potassium absorption [36]. After small bowel resection, colonic bacterial adaptation occurs and SCFA production and absorption increases [37]. Consequently, carbohydrate-derived energy can be salvaged in short bowel patients with even partial colonic preservation [18, 37-40]. The colon is therefore very beneficial not only for fluid and electrolyte conservation, but also for the salvage of malabsorbed energy substrates in short bowel patients [17-19, 37-41].

Adaptive function of the small intestine

After intestinal resection, the process of colonic bacterial flora adaptation during oral feeding continues for a number of weeks [37]. A decrease in stool fluid output is therefore seen following intestinal resection, after the reestablishment of colonic continuity when oral/enteral feeding is implemented [42]. This is not an argument against late, as opposed to early, intestinal adaptation [43]. The intestinal "hyper" adaptive process, which mainly depends on the presence of foods in the gut lumen, should not be diminished by the "hypo" adaptive process secondary to systemic malnutrition and/or food deprivation in the gut lumen [44-47]. The fact that significant small bowel adaptation is difficult to demonstrate in humans [42] does not rule out its clinical relevance. Indeed in the small bowel it has been demonstrated that there is a *functional* increase in the absorption of amino acids, glucose, sodium, water [48], calcium [49], cholesterol and vitamin B12 [50] months to years after small bowel resection. Furthermore, we recently demonstrated that hyperphagia [39] is adaptive during the long-term follow up of short-gut patients and that the increase in protein absorption was correlated with remaining small bowel length but not with oral intake [51]. The role of gut hormones and growth factors may in future offer further therapeutic options [52, 53]. These factors will have to demonstrate clear cut benefits over specific intestinal trophic nutrients, such as SCFAs and glutamine [53-55].

Consequences of intestinal resection

Intestinal failure

Intestinal resection reduces absorption of nutrients and is associated with a watery diarrhoea leading to increased losses of fluid, mineral and micronutrients. The severity of the malabsorption syndrome following intestinal resection depends on the extent, site and integrity of the intestinal remnant. Specific contributors to the severity of the malabsorption syndrome following short bowel resection are accelerated gastric emptying, reduced small bowel transit time, gastric acid hypersecretion, loose intercellular junctions in the jejunum, and loss of the unique function of the ileum. Other factors are mineral and micronutrient deficiencies such as potassium, magnesium, calcium, D, K, B1, B12 vitamins and zinc, which impair optimal function of the small intestine; antibiotic therapy may impair the salvage of fluid and nutrients from the colon. Short bowel patients with a small bowel remnant length of less than 150 cm are at high risk of weight loss, dehydration, and severe malnutrition. Indeed in 124 short bowel patients with non-malignant disease, parenteral nutrition (PN)-dependency was observed in 53% [44-62] and 45% [35-55] of cases at one and five years, respectively [11]. In the opinion of the author, it is better to correct, or avoid malnutrition through intravenous nutrition until full nutritional autonomy is obtained, rather than observing failure of oral nutrition followed by malnutrition.

Net digestive balances

Methods of performing balance studies have been summarized [10] and many balance studies have been published in patients with short bowel [19, 39, 41, 44, 56-58].

Non-oral nutritional autonomy (PN-dependency) has to be viewed as an isolated fluid electrolyte negative balance which may or may not be associated with a negative energy balance [56]. Fluid/electrolyte negative balances are observed in patients with a small bowel remnant length of less than 200 cm in 13% and 33% of cases with (n = 31) and without (n = 40) a colonic remnant, respectively [17]. A negative fluid-electrolyte balance is usually rapidly obvious (hours to days) and needs urgent treatment. Negative energy balance is usually a more prolonged and subtle event (weeks to months); it needs to be documented when starting, or changing the mode of nutritional support.

Net fluid electrolyte balance

Fluid losses from a stoma or as diarrhoea must be documented in short bowel patients. Losses range from up to 12,000 ml a day (duodenostomy) to a normal stool output (less than 300 g a day). Stool ionic losses can be estimated from the ouput and change dramatically from an end-enterostomy (similar to the ionic concentration of plasma) [28, 32] to a colostomy or a diarrhoea output where the proportion of colon resected is positively and negatively correlated to the sodium/chloride and potassium concentrations respectively [19] (table I). The risk for potassium depletion in end-enterostomy is greater in patients with a jejunal length remnant of less than 50 cm [56]. Potassium depletion is secondary to hyperaldosteronism due to water-sodium depletion associated with metabolic alkalosis and increased urinary potassium losses [41].

Net negative water/sodium balance was always observed in end-enterostomy patients with a jejunal length remnant of less than 100 cm, and rarely in those with a jejunal length of between 100 and 150 cm [56]. In patients with a colon remnant, the faecal potassium losses are associated with increased bicarbonate losses and a tendency to metabolic acidosis is not always compensated for by increased colonic production and absorption of acetate (this SCFA entering blood give an equimolar production of bicarbonate). Magnesium deficiency is very common in short bowel patients [10]. It may induce a 25% potassium depletion with increased extracellular water and oedema [59], and hypocalcaemia not responsive to vitamin D, but responsive to magnesium salts and/or the active metabolite (1alpha) of vitamin D [60].

Table I. Volume and osmotic constituents of proximal jejunal, mid-intestinal, lower ileum, mid-colon and terminal colon fluids

	Proximal-enterostomy	Mid-enterostomy	Ileum-enterostomy	50% colon*	100% colon*
Volume: l/d	6.0-4.0	3.0-1.5	1.0-0.5	2.0-1.0	1.0-0.5
Na^+	80-100	100-120	100-120	50-70	20-40
Cl^-	80-100	70-90	70-100	30-50	10-30
K^+	5-10	5-10	5-10	30-70	70-90
HCO_3	10-20	20-40	20-40	30-60	50-90

* 50% or 100% colon left with more than 100 cm ileal resection. Ionic concentrations are given in mosm/l. Data are adapted for short bowel patients from [19, 28, 68].

Net energy balance

Measurement of energy balance needs a bomb calorimeter and is recorded usually as net energy balance (intake-output), but can also be expressed as percentage of intake (intake-output/intake) [39, 56-58]. Energy balance in short bowel patients may range from – zero to normal (95% of intake). Endogenous losses may explain some rare negative energy balances [56]. In 15 short bowel patients with an end-enterostomy and a jejunal remnant length of 90 cm (range 25-140 cm), the patients ingested a diet which represented 1.8 fold their basal energy expenditure (BEE) and their net digestive absorption was 44% (range – 10% – 75%) of intake [56]. In ten short bowel patients with a small bowel remnant length of 75 cm (range, 0-200 cm) and a remnant colon length of 67% (range, 0-100%) the patients adapted to a hypercaloric, hyperprotein diet, which represented 2.5 fold their BEE, to compensate for increased faecal losses with output of 1,400 g (range, 300-3,800 g) per day; this hyperphagia does not seem to have impaired their net digestive absorption which was 67% (range 41%-85%) of intake. The higher net digestive absorption of carbohydrates compared with fat and protein suggested salvage of colonic carbohydrates [39]. A comparison between these two types of patients (table II) indicated a 50% difference in net energy balance when expressed as a % of BEE, from 0.8 fold the BEE in end-enterostomy patients to 1.7 fold the BEE in patients with a colon remnant [39, 56].

Table II. Net energy balance in short bowel patients

	End-enterostomy[a]	Jejuno(ileo)colonic anastomosis[b]
Oral intake: Kcal/d	2,500 (900-4,800)	3100 (1,700-4,500)
Faecal losses: Kcal/d	1,400 (550-2,700)	970 (340-1,600)
Coefficient of absorption: %	44 (−10-75)	67 (41-85)
Net absorption: Kcal/d	1,100 (−200-2,800)	2,130 (750-3,500)
Net absorption in % of BEE	0.80 (−0.2-2.0)	1.50 (0.55-3.3)

a (15 patients) and b (10 patients) data calculated from [56 and 39] respectively.
In a and b the remnant small bowel lengths were 90 (range, 25-140) cm of jejunum and 75 (0-200) cm respectively. For b, ileum was 15 (10-30) cm in four cases and absent in the 6 other cases; percentage of remnant colon was 67 (0-100) %. BEE = basal energy expenditure; BEE × 1.3 fold can estimate total EE for sedentary people. Urinary energy losses were measured at 300 Kcal in b patients without PN, a value which should be added to net digestive energy balance, for assessment of total body losses.

Clinical definition of severe intestinal failure

A consensus definition of severe intestinal failure is pending in the literature. Clinical features associated with severe intestinal failure are negative balances with a need for equilibrium or positive balances, provided by either a full PN regimen or water and mineral (sodium/potassium/magnesium) parenteral supplements [3, 10]. Patients in whom a definitive HPN is needed can be classified as having severe and irreversible intestinal failure. In our population of 124 short bowel patients, 48% were PN-dependent and PN treatment in this subgroup lasted for 44 (1-160) months [11]. It is worth noting that 24% of the non PN-dependent patients recovered full oral nutritional autonomy after 3 (1,5-46) months of PN. Our patients were able and encouraged to take free oral alimentation, and with subsequent hyperphagia [35] presumably developed their maximal absorptive capacity [36]. In contrast to other data [42], this finding indicates that intestinal adaptation may occur following the months after resection. In non PN-dependent patients, weaning was achieved within 24 months of PN in 95% [11]. This 2-year PN duration may serve as a guide to classify short bowel patients into reversible, or irreversible intestinal failure groups [61].

In recent actuarial data [11], PN-dependency was related to small bowel remnant length and to the three main circuit types of anastomosis [15-17]. Indeed, small bowel lengths associated with a significant decrease in PN-dependency rate changed according to the type of anastomosis. It was 100 cm in short bowel patients type I; a finding in accordance with the 100 cm remnant length reported to be associated with positive water-energy balance with oral feeds only and subsequent weaning off from PN [15-17, 56]. Cutoff values for type II and III were much lower: 65 and 30 cm respectively, attesting to an energy-sparing effect from oral feeds due to the presence in intestinal continuity of either a colon remnant or an ileum remnant and the ileocaecal valve [17-19, 37-39]. Interestingly, adult patients with short bowel types II/III with small bowel lengths over 50-70/30-35 cm respectively were in non-actuarial studies reported as non PN-dependent patients [15-17, 62].

Biochemical assessment of severe intestinal failure

In animal models, enterocytes specifically produce systemic citrulline from glutamine and ornithine, an amino acid not incorporated into proteins [63]. Citrulline production depends on the enzyme pyrroline-5-carboxylate synthase, which is located predominantly in enterocytes [64]. Circulating citrulline is then metabolized into arginine by the kidney [64]. We recently demonstrated in 52 short bowel patients without severe renal failure a significantly lower post-absorptive plasma citrulline than in 57 controls (40 vs 20 umol/l) [65], an observation which has been made in rats with intestinal resection [66]. In our study, multivariate analysis indicated that citrulline concentration was related only to small bowel length ($r^2 = 0.75$) either measured peroperatively, or indirectly with an opisometer [51, 65]. These data suggest that post-absorptive plasma citrulline concentration is a specific biochemical marker of the enterocyte mass. It may serve to assess the severity of intestinal failure. Further research is needed in this field.

Complications of intestinal resection

Peptic ulcer, cholelithiasis, renal stones and D-lactic acid encephalopathy are known complications of the short bowel syndrome [3, 10, 17]. The two last complications are only seen in patients having a colon remnant [17]. The D-lactic acid encephalopathy is due to fermented malabsorbed carbohydrates producing D-lactate and absorption of this metabolite. It can be facilitated by B1 deficiency and induced by antibiotics that affect the colonic bacterial flora [67].

Management of intestinal failure due to intestinal resection

Nutrition and drug treatment

Current treatment is HPN, which has been recently reviewed [3-5]. Two recent comprehensive reviews dealt with enteral feeding recommendations and drug treatments which increase absorption and reduce high losses of short bowel patients at the three evolutive stages following an intestinal resection [3, 10]. The author shares the opinions expressed in these reviews [68, 69].

Alternative treatment to HPN for irreversible intestinal failure

For short bowel patients with severe and irreversible intestinal failure, alternative options to home-PN should be considered [3, 10, 14, 43], such as trophic factors that include combination of growth hormone, glutamine and a modified diet [52], surgical intestinal reconstructions such as intestinal loop lengthening in children [43, 62, 70], or jejunal loop reversal in adults [62, 66, 71, 72], or small bowel transplantation [14, 62, 74]. At present transplantation should be reserved as a life saving procedure when HPN is impossible, or has become associated with liver failure [43, 68]. These alternative treatments should be done in tertiary care centres [43, 62, 70-74].

References

1. Fleming CR, Remington M. Intestinal failure. In: Hill GI, ed. *Nutrition and the surgical patient*. Clinical Surgery International. Edinburgh: Churchill Livingstone, 1981: 219-35.
2. Messing B, Hébuterne X. Indications of home artificial nutrition. European Society for Enteral and Parenteral Nutrition. XIX Congress Educational Book, Amsterdam, 1997.
3. Jeejeebhoy KN. Small bowel failure: causes and current treatment options. In: Grant DR, Wood RFM, eds. *Small bowel transplantation*. London: Edward Arnold, 1994: 1-8.
4. Messing B. Home parenteral nutrition. In: Payne-James J, Grimble G, D Silk D, eds. *Artificial nutrition in clinical practice*. London: Edward Arnold, 1994: 365-79.
5. Messing B. Audit of adult home parenteral long term feeders: a view from France. *Nutrition* 1996; 12: 825-6.

6. Van Gossum A, Bakker H, De Francesco A, Ladefoged K, Leon-Sanz M, Messing B, et al. Home parenteral nutrition in adults: a multicentre survey in Europe in 1993 ESPEN-Home Artificial Nutrition Working Group. *Clin Nutr* 1996; 15: 53-9.
7. Messing B, Barnoud D, Beau P, Bornet JL, Chambrier C, Di Constanzo J, et al. Bilan 1993-1995 de la nutrition parentérale à domicile en centres agréés chez l'adulte en France. *Gastroenterol Clin Biol* 1997, in press.
8. Howard L, Ament M, Fleming CR, Shike M, Steiger E. Current use and clinical outcome of home parenteral and enteral nutrition therapies in the United States. *Gastroenterology* 1995; 109: 355-65.
9. Messing B, Lémann M, Landais P, Gouttebel MC, Gérard-Boncompain M, Saudin F, et al. Prognosis of patients with nonmalignant chronic intestinal failure receiving long-term home parenteral nutrition. *Gastroenterology* 1995; 108: 1005-15.
10. Nightingale JMD. Clinical problems of a short bowel and their treatment. *Proc Nutr Soc* 1994; 53: 373-91.
11. Messing B, Crenn P, Beau P, Matuchansky C, Rambaud JC. Parenteral nutrition dependence in adult short bowel syndrome patients. *Gastroenterology* 1996; 110 (Suppl) Abstract 346.
12. Blatchford GJ, Thompson JS, Rikkers LF. Intestinal resection in adults and causes and consequences. *Dig Surg* 1989; 6: 57-61.
13. Grosfeld JL, Rescoria FJ, West KW. Short bowel syndrome in infancy and chilhood: analysis of survival in 60 patients. *Am J Surg* 1986; 151: 41-6.
14. Goulet OJ, Ricour C. The short bowel syndrome. In: Buts JP, Sokal EM, eds. *Management of digestive and liver disorders in infants and children*. Elsevier, 1993: 307-18.
15. Gouttebel MC, Saint-Aubert B, Astre C, Joyeux H. Total parenteral nutrition needs in different types of short bowel syndrome. *Dig Dis Sci* 1986; 31: 718-23.
16. Carbonnel F, Cosnes J, Chevret S, Beaugerie L, Ngo Y, Malafosse M, et al. The role of anatomic factors in nutritional autonomy after extensive small bowel resection. *J Parent Enteral Nutr* 1996; 20: 275-80.
17. Nightingale JMD, Lennard-Jones JE, Gertner DJ, Wood SR, Bartram CI. Colonic preservation reduces need for parenteral therapy, increases incidence of renal stones, but does not change high prevalence of gall stones in patients with a short bowel. *Gut* 1992; 33: 1493-7.
18. Nordgaard I, Hansen BS, Mortensen PB. Colon as a digestive organ in patients with short bowel. *Lancet* 1994; 343: 373-6.
19. Cummings JH, James WPT, Wiggins HS. Role of the colon in ileal-resection diarrhea. *Lancet* 1973; i: 344-7.
20. Nightingale JMD, Bartram CI, Lennard-Jones JE. Length of residual small bowel after partial resection: correlation betweeen radiographic and surgical measurements. *Gastrointest Radiol* 1991; 16: 305-6.
21. Malagelada JR. The gut response to a meal and its hormonal control. In: Bouchier IAD, Allan RN, Hodgson HJF, Keighley MRB, eds. *Gastroenterology; clinical science and practice*. London: WB Saunders, 1993, volume 1: 369-85.
22. Nightingale JMD, Kamm MA, van der Sijp JRM, Walker ER, Mather SJ, Britton KE, et al. Disturbed gastric emptying in the short bowel syndrome. Evidence for "a colonic brake". *Gut* 1993; 34: 1171-6.
23. Phillips SF, Quigley EMM, Kumar D, Kamath PS. Motility of the ileocolonic junction. *Gut* 1988; 29: 390-406.
24. Fich A, Staedman CJ, Phillips SF, Camilleri M, Brown ML, Haddad AC, et al. Ileocolonic transit does not change after righ hemicolectomy. *Gastroenterology* 1992; 103: 794-9.
25. Lin HC, Zhao XT, Wang L. Jejunal brake: inhibition of intestinal transit by fat in the proximal small intestine. *Dig Dis Sci* 1996; 41: 326-9.
26. Spiller RC, Trotman IF, Higgins BE, Ghatei MA, Grimble CK, Lee YC, et al. The ileal brake-inhibition of jejunal motility after ileal fat perfusion in man. *Gut* 1984; 25: 365-74.

27. Mahé S, Messing B, Thuillier F, Tomé D. Digestion of bovine milk proteins in patients with a high jejunostomy. *Am J Clin Nutr* 1991; 54: 534-9.
28. Fordtran JS, Locklear TW. Ionic constituents and osmolality of gastric and small- intestinal fluids after eating. *Am J Dig Dis* 1966; 11: 503-21.
29. Christopher NL, Bayless TM. Role of the small bowel and colon in lactose-induced diarrhea. *Gastroenterology* 1971; 60: 845-52.
30. Newton CR, Gonvers JJ, McIntyre PB, Preston DM, Lennard-Jones JE. The effect of different types of drinks on fluid and electrolyte losses from a jejunostomy. *J R Soc Med* 1985; 78: 27-34.
31. Read NW. Intestinal transport of fluid and electrolytes (physiology and pathophysiology). In: Bouchier IAD, Allan RN, Hodgson HJF, Keighley MRB, eds. *Gastroenterology; clinical science and practice*. London: WB Saunders, 1993, volume 1: 447-59.
32. Arrambide KA, Santa Ana CA, Schiller LR, Little KH, Santangelo WC, Fordtran JS. Loss of absorptive capacity for sodium chloride as a cause of diarrhea following partial ileal and right colon resection. *Dig Dis Sci* 1989; 34: 193-201.
33. Hoffman AF, Poley JR. Role of bile acid malabsorption in the pathogenesis of diarrhea and steatorrhea in patients with ileal resection. I. Response to cholestyramine or replacement of dietary long-chain triglycerides by medium-chain triglycerides. *Gastroenterology* 1972; 62: 918-34.
34. Phillips SF, Giller J. The contribution of the colon to electrolyte and water conservation in man. *J Lab Clin Med* 1973; 81: 733-46.
35. Debongnie JC, Phillips SF. Capacity of the colon to absorb fluid. *Gastroenterology* 1978; 74: 698-703.
36. Ruppin H, Bar-Meir S, Soergel KH, Wood CM, Schmitt MG Jr: Absorption of short chain fatty acids by the colon. *Gastroenterology* 1980; 78: 1500-7.
37. Briet F, Flourié B, Achour L, Maurel M, Rambaud JC, Messing B. Bacterial adaptation in patients with short bowel and colon in continuity. *Gastroenterology* 1995; 109: 1446-53.
38. Royall D, Wolever TM, Jeejeebhoy KN. Clinical significance of colonic fermentation. *Am J Gastroenterol* 1990; 85: 1307-12.
39. Messing B, Pigot F, Rongier M, Morin MC, Ndeindoum U, Rambaud JC. Intestinal absorption of free oral alimentation in very short bowel syndrome. *Gastroenterology* 1991; 100: 1502-8.
40. Nordgaard I, Hansen BS, Mortensen PB. Importance of colonic support for energy absorption as small-bowel failure proceeds. *Am J Clin Nutr* 1996; 64: 222-31.
41. Ladefoged K, Olgaard K. Fluid and electrolyte absorption and renin angiotensin-aldosterone axis in patients with severe short bowel syndrome. *Gastroenterology* 1979; 14: 729-35.
42. Cosnes J, Carbonnel F, Beaugerie L, Ollivier JM, Parc R, Gendre JP, Le Quintrec Y. Functional adaptation after extensive small bowel resection in humans. *Eur J Gastroenterol Hepatol* 1994; 6: 197-202.
43. Powell-Tuck J. Management of gut failure: a physician's view. *Lancet* 1994; 344: 1061-4.
44. Levy E, Frileux P, Sandrucci S, Ollivier JM, Masini JP, Cosnes J, et al. Continuous enteral nutrition during the early adaptive stage of the short bowel syndrome. *Br J Surg* 1988; 75: 549-53.
45. Levine CM, Deren JD, Yezdimer E. Small bowel resection; oral intake is the stimulus for hyperplasia. *Dig Dis Sci* 1976; 34: 709-15.
46. Feldman EJ, Dowling RH, McNaughton J, Peters TJ. Effect of oral versus intravenous nutrition on intestinal adaptation after small bowel resection in the dog. *Gastroenterology* 1976; 70: 712-9.
47. Biasco G, Callegari C, Lami F, Minarini A, Miglioli M, Barbara L. Intestinal morphological changes during oral refeeding in a patient previously treated with total parenteral nutrition for small bowel resection. *Am J Gastroenterol* 1984; 79: 585-8.
48. Dowling RH, Booth CC. Functional compensation after small bowel resection in man. Demonstration by direct measurement. *Lancet* 1966; ii: 146-7.
49. Gouttebel MC, Saint-Aubert B, Colette C, Monnier LH, Joyeux H. Intestinal adaptation in patients with short bowel syndrome. Measurement by calcium absorption. *Dig Dis Sci* 1989; 34: 709-15.

50. Koivisto P, Miettinen TA. Adaptation of cholesterol and bile acid metabolism and vitamin B12 absorption in the long-term follow-up after partial ileal bypass. *Gastroenterology* 1986; 90: 984-90.
51. Crenn P, Matuchansky C, Messing B. Clinical and biochemical modelization of post surgical intestinal failure in human adults. *Clin Nutr* 1997; 16: 133-5.
52. Byrne TA, Persinger RL, Young LS, Ziegler TS, Wilmore DW. A new treatment for patients with short-bowel syndrome: growth hormone, glutamine and a modified diet. *Ann Surg* 1995; 222: 243-55.
53. Foltzer-Jourdaine C, Raul F. Facteurs de croissance intestinaux. *Nutr Clin Metabol* 1996; 10: 325-35.
54. Fürst P, Stehle P. Glutamine and glutamine containing peptides. In: Cynober LA, ed. *Amino acid metabolism and therapy in health and nutritional disease.* London: CRC Press Boca Raton, 1995: 373-83.
55. Seal CJ, Reynolds CK. Nutritional implications of gastrointestinal and liver metabolism in ruminants. *Nutr Res Rev* 1993; 6: 185-208.
56. Nightingale JMD, Lennard-Jones JE, Walker ER, Farthing MJG. Jejunal efflux in short bowel syndrome. *Lancet* 1990; 336: 765-8.
57. Woolf GM, Miller C, Kurian R, Jeejeebhoy KN. Diet for patients with a short bowel. High fat or high carbohydrate? *Gastroenterology* 1983; 84: 823-8.
58. Woolf GM, Miller C, Kurian R, Jeejeebhoy KN. Nutritional absorption in short bowel syndrome. Evaluation of fluid, calorie, and divalent cation requirements. *Dig Dis Sci* 1987; 32: 8-15.
59. Shils M. Experimental production of magnesium deficiency in man. *Ann NY Acad Sci* 1969; 162: 847-56.
60. Ducreux M, Messing B, De Vernejoule MC, Bouhnik Y, Miravet L, Rambaud JC. Calcemic response to magnesium or 1-alpha-hydroxy-cholecalciferol treatment in intestinal hypomagnesemia. *Gastroenterol Clin Biol* 1991; 15: 805-11.
61. Ingham Clark CL, Lear PA, Wood S, Lennard-Jones JE, Wood RFM. Potential candidates for small bowel transplantation. *Br J Surg* 1992; 79: 676-9.
62. Thompson JS, Langnas AN, Pinch LW, Kaufman S, Quigley EMM, Vanderhoof JA. Surgical approach to short bowel syndrome. Experience in a population of 160 patients. *Ann Surg* 1995; 222: 600-7.
63. Windmueller HG, Spaaeth AE. Source and fate of circulating citrulline. *Am J Physiol* 1981; 241: E473-80.
64. Wakabayashi Y, Yamada E, Hasegawa T, Yamada R. Enzymological evidence for the indispensability of small intestine in the synthesis of arginine from glutamate: I Pyrollone-5-carboxylate synthase. *Arch Biochem Biophys* 1991; 291: 1-8.
65. Crenn P, Coudray-Lucas C, Cynober L, Darmaun D, Messing B. Plasma concentrations of amino acids with a predominant site of intestinal metabolism. *Gastroenterology* 1996; 110 (Suppl): A79666.
66. Wakabayashi Y, Yamada E, Yoshida T, Takahashi H. Effect of intestinal resection and arginine-free diet on rat physiology. *Am J Physiol* 1995; 269: G313-8.
67. Flourié B, Messing B, Bismuth E, Etanchaud F, Thuillier F, Rambaud JC. Acidose D lactique et encéphalopathie au cours d'un syndrome du grêle court à l'occasion d'un traitement antibiotique. *Gastroenterol Clin Biol* 1990; 14: 596-8.
68. Messing B, Pigot F. Diététique des syndromes de grêle court chez l'adulte. I: Bases physiopathologiques. *Cah Nutr Diet* 1989; 24: 306-10.
69. Pigot F, Messing B. Diététique des syndromes de grêle court chez l'adulte. I: Bases physiopathologiques. *Cah Nutr Diet* 1989; 24: 395-9.
70. Quigley EMM. Small intestinal transplantation: reflections on an evolving approach to intestinal failure. *Gastroenterology* 1996; 110: 2009-12.
71. Georgeson K, Halpin D, Figueroa R, Vincente Y, Hardin W. Sequencial intestinal lengthening procedures for refractory short bowel syndrome. *J Pediatr Surg* 1994; 29: 316-21.
72. Pigot F, Messing B, Chaussade S, Pfeiffer A, Pouliquen X, Jian R. Severe short bowel syndrome with a surgically reversed small bowell segment. *Dig Dis Sci* 1990; 35: 137-44.

73. Panis Y, Messing B, Rivet P, Coffin B, Hautefeuille P, Matuchansky C, *et al*. Segmental reversal of the small bowel as an alternative of intestinal transplantation in patients with short bowel syndrome. *Ann Surg* 1997; 225: 356-61.
74. Grant D. Current results of intestinal transplantation. *Lancet* 1996; 347: 1801-3.

Evidence-Based Clinical Gastroenterology.
M.J.G. Farthing, J.J. Misiewicz, eds. John Libbey Eurotext, Paris © 1997, pp. 41-54.

Management of primary biliary cirrhosis

P.L.M. Jansen

Division of Hepatology and Gastroenterology, University Hospital Groningen, The Netherlands

Summary

Primary biliary cirrhosis is a slowly progressive cholestatic liver disease with autoimmune features. Antimitochondrial antibodies are detected in the serum of 95 percent of patients. The antibodies are directed against the E2 component of the pyruvate dyhydrogenase complex on the inner mitochondrial membrane. Fatigue, pruritus and bone pain are the most troublesome complaints which affect the quality of life of these patients. Ursodeoxycholic acid therapy has been shown to improve laboratory values, symptoms and in some trials also the liver histology. An influence on survival has not been proved. New trials are being conducted where ursodeoxycholic acid is combined with immunosuppressive, antiinflammatory or antifibrotic drugs. Prognostic models have been developed that help in the planning of liver transplantation. As primary biliary cirrhosis probably can recur in the transplanted liver, its clinical relevance in the long-run needs to be assessed.

The first description of primary biliary cirrhosis is ascribed to Thomas Addison and William Gull in a paper published in 1851 [1]. These authors grasped two essential features of this desease, when they described six patients with jaundice, vitiligo, xanthomas, cholestasis and autoimmunity.

Pathogenesis

The term primary biliary cirrhosis (PBC) is a misnomer because fibrosis is a late phenomenon. The disease results from a chronic "non-suppurative" inflammation of the small and medium-sized bile ducts. There are several reasons to suspect that this initial lesion is immunologically mediated with an emphasis on autoimmunity. However, there are some interesting findings and speculations to suggest that allogenic stimuli may initiate the disease and that the disease results from an inherited abnormality of immunoregulation. The discussion here is not unlike the one in Crohn's disease. The disease may be triggered by exposure to atypical mycobacteria, or to certain mutants of enterobacteriaceae. Sera from PBC patients have been shown to react with membranes from these microorganisms [2-4]. Abnormalities of bile acid metabolism, drug metabolism and glutathione metabolism have also been proposed [5-8]. Although the discussion concerning initiation of PBC is still very hypothetical, the relation between PBC and autoimmunity and defects of immunoregulation in this disease, are more firmly established.

Like all autoimmune diseases, PBC predominantly occurs in females. The serum immunoglobulins, particularly the IgM fraction, are elevated; there is an abundance of auto-antibodies; the blood contains activated T and B cells and the liver shows lymphoid aggregates and granulomas. There is T-cell mediated bile duct destruction and HLA class-II expression on the bile duct epithelium. Circulating auto-antibodies include antimitochondrial and antinuclear antibodies, such as antibodies against the nuclear membrane, antihistone antibodies, antiribonucleoprotein-antigen antibodies and anticentromere antibodies. The antigens with which the antimitochondrial antibodies (AMA) react have been characterized using modern cloning techniques: they include components of the pyruvate dehydrogenase complex (PDC) on the inner mitochondrial membrane, the most important of these are directed against the E2 component of PDC [9, 10]. These AMA antibodies are present in 95 percent of patients with PBC and their specificity is 98 percent. Whether they play a pathogenic role is debated. In PBC patients an aberrant expression of a protein with PDC-E2 immunoreactivity has been observed in the biliary epithelium [11]. This is not due to an increased expression of PDC-E2 mRNA [12]. Whether this protein is a bacterial product with PDC-E2 cross-reactivity, or an aberrant protein of ductular or hepatocellular origin, is at present unknown.

AMA levels are not correlated with disease activity and do not predict disease progression, response to ursodeoxycholic acid therapy or outcome of liver transplantation [13, 14]. A small fraction of patients has all the clinical, laboratory and histological features of PBC with the exception that they are AMA-negative [15]. The clinical course of this subgroup of patients is similar to that of AMA-positive patients [16].

PBC is associated with a host of autoimmune diseases such as vitiligo, autoimmune thyroiditis, Sjögren's syndrome, rheumatoid arthritis, scleroderma, CREST syndrome, lichen planus, systemic lupus erythematosus, jejunal villous atrophy, ulcerative colitis and autoimmune gastritis.

Metabolic consequences

Immune-mediated bile duct destruction inevitably leads to cholestasis. The parenchymal damage present in late stage PBC is most probably the consequence of accumulation of toxic products, in particular bile salts. Accumulation of bile salts leads to mitochondrial dysfunction, feathery degeneration of hepatocytes, apoptosis of hepatocytes and bile duct epithelium and enhanced expression of HLA class II and class I molecules.

Cholestasis is responsible for the many extrahepatic metabolic problems in PBC, such as hepatic osteodystrophy with disabling osteoporosis, accumulation of lipids with xanthelasmata, fatty streaks and xanthomas, and malnutrition. In the gut bile acids bind endotoxins. In more advanced stages of the disease, portal endotoxaemia may add to the liver injury as lipopolysaccharide (LPS) stimulates the production of tumour necrosis factor α (TNFα) and interleukin-6 (IL-6) by Küpffer cells. These and other LPS-stimulated cytokines may be important for the initiation of liver fibrosis as they stimulate the transformation of hepatic stellate cells into collagen-producing myofibroblasts. TNFα is also an important initiating factor in liver regeneration and therefore bile acid-induced apoptosis and TNFα-mediated regeneration and fibrosis are key elements in the pathogenesis of liver cirrhosis.

Chronic cytokine production may also contribute to the malnutrition seen in advanced disease: TNFα depletes adipocytes and IL-6 inhibits the hepatic production or release of insulin-like growth factor-I, an important anabolic hormone [17]. In addition, there are disturbances of vitamin D metabolism although the prevailing bone disease is osteoporosis rather than osteomalacia [18]. Vitamin K absorption is decreased, with clotting factor abnormalities as a consequence. Later in the disease, when hepatocellular dysfunction becomes dominant, blood clotting abnormalities become resistant to vitamin K. There are derangements of lipid metabolism with increased levels of HDL-cholesterol and lipoprotein X, but atherosclerotic heart disease is uncommon in these patients [19]. Altered bile composition leads to an increased incidence of gallstones in patients with PBC. Pruritus is probably not due to bile acids, but may be centrally mediated [20, 21]. Fatigue may also be CNS-mediated [22, 23].

Prevalence

PBC has been estimated to occur with a prevalence of about 20-150 cases per 100,000 population [24]. Some high incidence areas have been described, but whether this is due to a particular local interest in the disease, or to a real difference in geographical distribution due to genetic or environemental factors, is uncertain [25].

Diagnosis

PBC is typically, but not exclusively, a disease of middle aged women. Fatigue and pruritus are the salient presenting features and remain the most disabling symptoms during the course of the disease. On physical examination the liver is initially enlarged. Jaundice, xanthomas, splenomegaly, spider naevi and ascites are late phenomena. Oesophageal varices may develop before liver cirrhosis becomes manifest as result of pre-sinusoidal portal hypertension [26]. Most patients are detected because of their symptoms, mostly fatigue or pruritus, or because of laboratory abnormalities. Increased alkaline phosphatase, or a positive antimitochondrial factor may be the only abnormalities observed during laboratory screening performed for some other reason. Most of these patients are asymptomatic, but eventually will develop symptoms [27, 28]. The salient laboratory abnormalities of

Bone disease

Osteoporosis is common in PBC, osteomalacia is rare. In a recent study about 35 percent of patients with PBC had osteoporosis to some degree. This is not due to lack of vitamin D or calcium. It is probably related to an increased bone resorption and suppressed osteoblast activity [18, 32-34]. The effects of vitamin D, calcium, calcitonin, oestrogens and ursodeoxycholic acid have been variable and usually disappointing [34, 35]. Biphosphonates have not been systematically studied in this condition. Regular exercise and administration of calcium and vitamin D supplements is the usual practical advice. Oestrogen supplementation, for example in a low transdermally administered dose, may be considered in post-menopausal women, although appropriate trials have not been done yet.

Accelerated bone loss is seen the first three months after liver transplantation [32]. A recent sudy showed that cyclic ethidronate does not prevent this [36]. Eventually bone loss stops and the bone mass may be restored to normal, 2-3 years after liver transplantation [32, 37].

Clotting abnormalities

Vitamin K deficiency is rare in this condition. Most physicians however treat their patients with oral vitamin K 10 mg per day. When despite this supplementation clotting abnormalities occur, this most likely is due to the progression of liver failure. Thrombocytopenia is frequent, not only because of hyperplenism, but also because of a high incidence of autoimmune thrombocytopenia. Blood clotting in PBC seems better preserved than in other liver diseases. A recent study showed that PBC patients at transplantation have a preserved capacity to generate thrombin and have a lower fibrinolytic activity than non-PBC liver transplantation candidates [38].

Nutritional status

The assessment of the nutritional status of liver cirrhosis patients is difficult. In advanced liver cirrhosis patients are frequently malnourished. The cause is multifactorial. Patients are sometimes prescribed impalatable diets with restrictions of fat, protein, fluids and salt. A fully nutritional diet with some diuretic or lactulose would be a more human approach. Salt and fluid restriction may become necessary only when severe ascites does not respond to diuretic therapy. Regular paracentesis may be preferable in this situation.

Patients with liver cirrhosis are anorexic and this may be parly due to impaired taste and olfactory perception [39]. Deficiency of zinc and magnesium may contribute to impaired taste. In addition, *foetor hepaticus* and Sjögren's syndrome are contributing factors. Zinc and magnesium can be supplemented.

Steatorrhoea, jejunal villous atrophy and pancreatic insufficiency may contribute to malnutrition. Hormonal derangements such as increased insulin-resistance and IGF-I deficiency also contribute to the malnourishment [40]. In case of steatorrhoea, pancreatic enzyme supplementation may be tried. Ursodeoxycholic acid therapy does not improve steatorrhoea, in fact UDCA impairs the ileal absorption of primary bile acids. Nutritional status is an underestimated risk factor with predictive power towards the outcome of liver transplantation [41].

Fatigue

There is no single drug yet available to treat fatigue in patients with liver cirrhosis. Fatigue seems to be particularly prominent in chronic cholestatic conditions like PBC and primary sclerosing cholangitis. Its cause is unknown. It may be related to deranged muscle metabolism with an increased energy expenditure per work load. Recent research indicates that fatigue may be a behavioural problem. A 5-hydroxytryptamine$_{1A}$- receptor agonist caused a return of activity score in cholestatic rats to normal [22, 23]. This suggests that fatigue in cholestatic conditions may be related to altered serotoninergic neurotransmission and that 5-HT$_{1A}$ receptor agonists may be able to reverse this. This opens a new and interesting venue for clinical exploration.

Pruritus

The cause of pruritus in cholestatic liver disease is still conjectural. It may be due to stimulation of peripheral nerve endings by certain compounds, bile acids or others, or to centrally-mediated alterations of neurotransmission. Cholestyramine is the most frequently used drug for this complaint. It is a bile acid-binding resin, but it also binds fat-soluble vitamins. Phenobarbital and rifampicin also decrease pruritus. These are inducers of some cytochrome P-450 and UDP-glucuronosyltransferase isoenzymes and their mode of action may be due to increased metabolism of bile acids, or related itch-producing compounds. In some studies, ursodeoxycholic was shown to relieve the itch, although initially it may aggravate pruritus. Pruritus may be centrally mediated and opiate-antagonists such as naloxone, its oral analogue naltrexone, or ondansetron, a 5-HT$_3$ serotonin receptor antagonist, induced relief of pruritus in cholestatic patients [20, 21, 42]. None of the treatments is entirely satisfactory and liver transplantation may eventually be indicated for severe relentless pruritus that has a negative influence on the quality of life.

Drugs under investigation at present

The natural history of PBC is well described (although long-term studies up to 10-15 years are still needed), and validated prognostic models are available [30, 31, 43, 44]. Therefore PBC seems a good subject for randomized controlled drug trials, where endpoints such as survival and delay of transplantation are studied. Unfortunately the pathogenesis of the disease is still obscure and this is reflected in the drugs that have been tried. These include antifibrotic and antiinflammatory drugs (d-penicillamine, colchicine), immunosuppressive drugs (corticosteroids, cyclosporine, methotrexate, chlorambucil) and a bile salt agonist/antagonist (ursodeoxycholic acid).

Table I lists the drugs that have been studied in randomized controlled trials since 1994. Single drug trials of colchicine, d-penicillamine, methotrexate, prednisolone and cyclosporin have been performed earlier and have either not yielded convincing results, or caused too many side effects, or both; d-penicillamine has been widely studied, but appears to be without effect; colchicine improved biochemical variables, but not symptoms, histology or survival; methotrexate has only been used in small trials and is known to cause pneumonitis; prednisolone causes osteopenia – particularly in PBC patients; and cyclosporin is nephrotoxic (summarized in [45]). In none of these trials have the side-effects outweighed the benefits.

Ursodeoxycholic acid has been the most widely studied drug. It is particularly attractive because it has almost no side effects, with the exception that initially pruritus can worsen. Ursodeoxycholic acid has been shown to reduce serum alkaline phosphatase and less often also the conjugated bilirubin. It has also been shown to decrease the IgM titre and the serum procollagen III peptide concentrations, a marker for liver fibrosis. Beneficial effects on liver histology were less consistent. In one study it delayed the time of transplantation. In general, patients seem to feel better while on ursodeoxycholic acid. This may be a psychological effect because of improvement of jaundice. For more promising combinations the outcome of trials with various drug combinations is awaited. A word of caution is necessary; for some of these trials patients who were already treated with ursodeoxycholic acid were selected. Physicians will be inclined to include in subsequent trials patients who had an unsatisfactory response to ursodeoxycholic acid alone. Thus a selection bias may be introduced by selecting a group of non- or poor-responders. It is better to include naive patients in these trials, but these are difficult to find, because most patients are treated nowadays with ursodeoxycholic acid from the time of diagnosis. Trial centres should therefore encourage physicians to include in treatment combination trials patients who already responded to urso therapy, to determine if further improvement is possible.

Liver transplantation

In many liver transplantation centres, in particular those of Northern Europe, PBC is a major indication. Since PBC is a slowly progressive disease with a more or less predictable course, timing of transplantation in PBC is less difficult than in some of the other chronic liver diseases. Timing is much helped by the predictive power of the serum bilirubin level, or by the more refined Mayo risk score, or by the Christensen model. Recent data from three large US transplantation centres showed that transplantation candidates with PBC are usually in Child-Pugh class B or C, their Mayo risk score is 7.3, 68 per cent have ascites, about half have encephalopathy, their nutritional status is "fair" and their serum bilirubin level is about 100 μmol/l [57]. The transplantation procedure seems to carry a reasonable risk, with a median blood loss of 2.2 litres and a median ICU stay of 3 days.

Table I. The outcome of drug trials in primary biliary cirrhosis

First author	Drugs	Urso dose mg/kg	Follow-up years	Patients n	Improvement of symptoms	Toxicity	Decrease of alk phos and/or CB	Improvement of histology	Influence on survival and/or time transplantation
Poupon [46]	urso vs plac	13-15	4	145	nt	-	+	+	+
Combes [47]	urso vs plac	10-12	2	151	+	-	+[1]	+[1]	-
Heathcote [48]	urso vs plac	14	2	222	-	-	+	+	-
Lindor [49]	urso vs plac	13-15	4 (2)	180	-	-	+	-	-
Eriksson [50]	urso vs plac	7.7	2 (4)	116	-	-	+	-	-
Ikeda [51]	urso + col vs urso	11.3	2	22	-	+	+	nt	nt
Poupon [52]	urso + col vs urso	13-15	2	74	-	-	-	-	nt
Leuschner [53]	urso + pred vs urso	10	3	29	-[2]	-	-[2]	+	nt
Wolfhagen [54]	urso + pred + aza vs urso	10	1	50	+	+	+	+	-
Gonzalez [55]	urso + mtx vs urso	10	4	25	-	-	-[2]	-[2]	nt
Lindor [56]	urso + mtx vs urso	13-15	2	32 vs 180	-	+	-[2]	-[2]	nt

1. In the Combes trial patient groups were stratified in four groups based on serum bilirubin levels and severity of liver histology, results were significant for the two groups with less severe disease.
2. In these trials no beneficial effect of the combination was seen but symptoms and/or laboratory values improved in both arms suggesting a beneficial effect due to ursodeoxycholic acid.
Abbreviations: urso, ursodeoxycholic acid; pla, placebo; mtx, methotrexate; pred, prednisolone; aza, azathioprine; alk phos, alkaline phosphatase; CB, conjugated bilirubin.

The retransplantation rate is about 10 per cent. Survival at one year is 85-90 per cent and 70-75 per cent at 5 years. Bone pain and fractures are important post-transplant complications in PBC patients, despite good self-perceived health and return to daily activities after transplantation [58].

Does PBC recur after transplantation?

Histologically recurrence of PBC is difficult to distinguish from chronic ductopenic rejection, viral or drug-induced liver disease. This has therefore been a controversial issue [59-63]. In addition to immunohistochemical evidence of disease recurrence [62], there are several studies that suggest histological recurrence [61, 63]. With some exceptions, these recurrences do not appear to have clinical consequences, but one wonders what will happen in the long-run with patients who have evidence of recurrence 5 years after transplantation. Slapak *et al.* studied the prevalence of biochemical and histological graft abnormalities 5 years after transplantation in 116 patients transplanted by the King's College/Cambridge group [61]. Thirty-three of these were transplanted for PBC. In 8 of these, PBC-like abnormalities were found. Four had liver function abnormalities. One of these patients died with stage 3 recurrent PBC at autopsy. In another 8 patients a picture of HCV-negative chronic hepatitis was seen. Whether or not this is related to PBC could not be ascertained. The effect of immunosuppression was studied by Dmitrewski *et al.* [63]. In Birmingham 27 patients were transplanted for PBC. In a randomized trial half were treated with cyclosporin and half with FK 506. Half of the patients on FK 506 developed histological evidence of recurrent PBC, two years after transplantation. This occurred in only one of 11 patients on cyclosporin. The conclusion was that immunosuppressive therapy may influence PBC recurrence after liver transplantation.

Conclusions

The message for the individual patient can be summarised as follows:
- patients with serum bilirubin below 34 µmol/l (2 mg/dl) are the best responders to drug therapy and can be treated with ursodeoxycholic acid, in a dose of 10-15 mg/kg;
- since the final answer to drug therapy is not yet known, it is better to include patients who fall into this category in one of the newer drug trials, comparing combinations of drugs *versus* ursodeoxycholic acid alone;
- patients with serum bilirubin above 34 µmol/l and/or ascites and/or bleeding varices and/or encephalopathy should be referred to a transplantation centre;
- patients with serum bilirubin above 100-150 µmol/l, a one-year life expectancy below 60-70 percent, and/or a Mayo risk score of 7.3 or higher, should be transplanted;
- patients with a poor quality of life because of intractable pruritus or extreme fatigue, are transplantation candidates.

References

1. Mistry P, Seymour CA. Primary biliary cirrhosis-from Thomas Addison to the 1990s. *Quart J Med* 1992; 82: 185-96.
2. Vilagut L, Pares A, Rodes J, Vila J, Vinas O, Gines A, Jimenez de Anta MT. Myocobacteria-related to the aetiopathogenesis of primary biliary cirrhosis? [letter]. *J Hepatol* 1996; 24: 125.
3. Berg PA, Klein R. Mycobacteria-related to the aetiopathogenesis of primary biliary cirrhosis? [letter]. *J Hepatol* 1995; 23: 103.
4. Stemerowicz R, Hopf U, Moller B, et al. Are antimitochondrial antibodies in primary biliary cirrhosis induced by R (rough) mutants of enterobacteriaceae? *Lancet* 1988; ii: 1166.
5. Davis MH, Elias E, Acharya S, et al. GSTM1 null polymorphism at the glutathione S-transferase M1 locus: phenotype and genotype studies in patients with primary biliary cirrhosis. *Gut* 1993; 345: 49-54.
6. Farinati F, Cardin R, Naccarato R, Floreani A. Cysteine and glutathione in the liver of patients with primary biliary cirrhosis [letter]. *J Hepatol* 1996; 25: 123.
7. Olomu AB, Vickers CR, Waring RH, et al. High incidence of poor sulfoxidation in patients with primary biliary cirrhosis. *N Engl J Med* 1988; 318: 1089.
8. Davies MH, Ngong JM, Pean A, Vickers CR, Waring RH, Elias E. Sulphoxidation and sulphation capacity in patients with primary biliary cirrhosis. *J Hepatol* 1995; 22: 551-60.
9. Gershwin ME, Mackay IR, Sturgess A, et al. Identification and specificity of a cDNA encoding the 70-kDa mitochondrial antigen recognised in primary biliary cirrhosis. *J Immunol* 1987; 138: 352-5.
10. Yeaman SJ, Fussey SPM, Danner DJ, et al. Primary biliary cirrhosis: identification of two major M2 mitochondrial autoantigens. *Lancet* 1988; i: 1067.
11. Tsuneyama K, Van de Water J, Leung PS, Cha S, Nakanuma Y, Kaplan M, De Lellis R, Coppel R, Ansari A, Gershwin ME. Abnormal expression of the E2 component of the pyruvate dehydrogenase complex on the luminal surface of biliary epithelium occurs before major histocompatibility complex class II and BB1/B7 expression. *Hepatology* 1995; 21: 1031-7.
12. Harada K, Van de Water J, Leung PS, Coppel RL, Nakanuma Y, Gershwin ME. *In situ* nucleic acid hybridization of pyruvate dehydrogenase complex-E2 in primary biliary cirrhosis: pyruvate dehydrogenase complex-E2 messenger RNA is expressed in hepatocytes but not in biliary epithelium. *Hepatology* 1997; 25: 27-32.
13. Van Norstrand MD, Malinchoc M, Lindor KD, Therneau TM, Gershwin ME, Leung PS, Dickson ER, Homburger HA. Quantitative measurement of autoantibodies to recombinant mitochondrial antigens in patients with primary biliary cirrhosis: relationship of levels autoantibodies to disease progression. *Hepatology* 1997; 25: 6-11.
14. Kim WR, Poterucha JJ, Jorgensen RA, Batts KP, Homburger HA, Dickson ER, Krom RAF, Wiesner RH, Lindor KD. Does antimitochondrial antibody status affect response to treatment in patients with primary biliary cirrhosis? Outcomes of ursodeoxycholic acid therapy and liver transplantation. *Hepatology* 1997; 26: 22-6.
15. O'Donohue J, Williams R. Antimitochondrial antibody and primary biliary cirrhosis: can there be one without the other? [editorial]. *J Hepatol* 1996; 25: 574-7.
16. Invernizzi P, Crosignani A, Battezzati PM, Covini G, De Valle G, Larghi A, Zuin M, Podda M. Comparison of the clinical features and clinical course of antimitochondrial antibody-positive and -negative primary biliary cirrhosis. *Hepatology* 1997; 25: 1090-5.
17. Guler HP, Zapf J, Froesch ER. Short-term metabolic effects of recombinant human insulin-like growth factor I in healthy adults. *N Engl Med J* 1987; 317: 137-40.
18. Diamond TH, Stiel D, Lunzer M, McDowall D, Eckstein RP, Posen S. Hepatic osteodystrophy. Static and dynamic bone histomorphometry and serum bone Gla-protein in 80 patients with chronic liver disease. *Gastroenterology* 1989; 96: 213-21.

19. Crippin JS, Lindor KD, Joergensen RA, et al. Hypercholesterolemia and atherosclerosis in primary biliary cirrhosis what is the risk? *Hepatology* 1992; 15: 858-62.
20. Bergasa NV, Talbot TL, Alling DW, Schmitt JM, Walker EC, Baker BL, Korenman JC, Park Y, Hoofnagle JH, Jones EA. A controlled trial of naloxone infusions for the pruritus of chronic cholestasis. *Gastroenterology* 1992; 102: 544-9.
21. Schworer H, Hartmann H, Ramadori G. Relief of cholestatic pruritus by a novel class of drugs: 5-hydroxytryptamine type 3 (5-HT3) receptor antagonists: effectiveness of ondansetron. *Pain* 1995; 6: 133-7.
22. Swain MG, Maric M. Improvement in cholestasis-associated fatigue with a serotonin receptor antagonist using a novel rat model of fatigue assessment. *Hepatology* 1997; 25: 291-4.
23. Jones EA, Yurdaydin C. Is fatigue associated with cholestasis mediated by altered central neurotransmission? *Hepatology* 1997; 25: 492-4.
24. Kaplan MM. Primary biliary cirrhosis. *N Engl J Med* 1996; 335: 1570-80.
25. Sherlock S, Dooley J. Primary biliary cirrhosis. In: Sherlock and Dooley, eds. *Diseases of the liver and biliary system* Oxford: Blackwell Science. 10th ed., 1997: 239-52.
26. Gores GJ, Wiesner RH, Dickson ER, et al. Prospective evaluation of oesophageal varices in primary biliary cirrhosis: development, Natural history and influence on survival. *Gastroenterology* 1989; 96: 1552.
27. Balasubramaniam K, Grambsch PM, Wiesner RH, et al. Diminished survival in asymptomatic primary biliary cirrhosis. A prospective study. *Gastroenterology* 1990; 98: 1567.
28. Metcalf JV, Mitchinson HC, Palmer JM, Jones DE, Bassendine MF, Jamsem OFW. Natural history of early primary biliary cirrhosis. *Lancet* 1996; 348: 1399-402.
29. Ludwig J, Dickson ER, Mac Donald GSA, et al. Staging of chronic non supparative destructive cholangitis (syndrome of primary biliary cirrhosis). *Virchows Arch Pathol Anatom* 1978; 379: 103.
30. Dickson ER, Grambsch PM, Fleming TR, Fisher LD, Langworthy A. Prognosis in primary biliary cirrhosis: model for decision making. *Hepatology* 1989: 101-7.
31. Christensen E, Altman DG, Neuberger J, De Stavola BL, Tygstrup N, Williams R. The PBC1 and PBC2 trial groups. Updating prognosis in primary biliary cirrhosis using a time-dependent Cox regression model. *Gastroenterology* 1993; 105: 1865-76.
32. Eastell R, Dickson ER, Hodgson SF, Wiesner RH, Porayko MK, Wahner HW, Cedel SL, Riggs BL, Krom RAF. Rates of vertebral bone loss before and after liver transplantation in women with primary biliary cirrhosis. *Hepatology* 1991; 14: 296-300.
33. Hodgson SF, Dickson ER, Wahner HW, Johnson KA, Mann KG, Riggs BL. Bone loss and reduced osteoblast function in primary biliary cirrhosis. *Ann Intern Med* 1985; 103: 855-60.
34. Mitchison HC, Malcolm AJ, Bassendine MF, James OFW. Metabolic bone disease in primary biliary cirrhosis at presentation. *Gastroenterology* 1988; 94: 463-70.
35. Lindor KD, Janes CH, Crippin JS, Jorgensen RA, Dickson ER. Bone disease in primary biliary cirrhosis: does ursodeoxycholic acid make a difference? *Hepatology* 1995; 21: 389-92.
36. Riemens SC, Oostdjik A, van Doormaal JJ, Thijn CJP, Drent G, Piers DA, Groen EWJ, Meerman L, Slooff MJH, Haagsma EB. Bone loss after liver transplantation is not prevented by cyclical etidronate, calcium and alphacalcidol. *Osteoporosis Int* 1996; 6: 213-8.
37. McDonald JA, Dunstan CR, Dillworth P, Sherbon K, Sheil AGR, Evans RA, McCaughan GW. Bone loss after transplantation. *Hepatology* 1991; 14: 613-9.
38. Segal H, Cottam S, Potter D, Hunt BJ. Coagulation and fibrinolysis in primary biliary cirrhosis compared with other liver disease and during orthotopic liver transplantation. *Hepatology* 1997; 25: 683-8.
39. Madden AM, Bradbury W, Morgan MY. Taste perception in cirrhosis: its relationship to circulating micronutrients and food preferences. *Hepatology* 1997; 26: 40-8.

40. Donaghy A, Ross R, Gimson A, Cwyfan Hughes S, Holly J, Williams R. Growth hormone, insulin-like growth factor-I, and insulin-like growth factor binding proteins 1 and 3 in chronic liver disease. *Hepatology* 1995; 21: 680-8.
41. Selberg O, Bottcher J, Pichlmayr R, Henkel E, Muller MJ. Identification of high- and low-risk patients before liver transplantation: a prospective cohort study of nutritional and metabolic parameters in 150 patients. *Hepatology* 1997; 25: 652-7.
42. Bergasa NV, Alling DW, Talbot TL, Swain MG, Yurdaydin C, Turner ML, Schmitt JM, et al. Effects of naloxone infusions in patients with the pruritus of cholestasis: a double-blind, randomized, controlled trial. *Ann Intern Med* 1995; 123: 161-7.
43. Grambsch PM, Dickson ER, Kaplan M, Lesage G, Fleming TR, Langworthy A. Extramural cross-validation of the Mayo primary biliary cirrhosis survival model establishes its generalizability. *Hepatology* 1989; 108: 46-50.
44. Bonsel GJ, Klompmaker IJ, V an't Veer F, Habbema JDF, Slooff MJH. Use of prognostic models for assessment of value of liver transplantation in primary biliary cirrhosis. *Lancet* 1990; 335: 493-7.
45. Poupon R, Poupon RE. Primary biliary cirrhosis. In: Zakim D, Boyer TD, eds. *Hepatology. A textbook of liver disease*. Philadelphia: Saunders, W.B. 3rd ed., 1996: 1329-65.
46. Poupon RE, Poupon R, Balkau B, and UDCA-PBC study group. Ursodiol for the long-term treatment of primary biliary cirrhosis. *N Engl J Med* 1994; 330: 1342-7.
47. Combes B, Carithers RL Jr, Maddrey WC, Lin D, McDonald MF, Wheeler DE, Eigenbrodt EH, Munoz SJ, Rubin R, Garcia Tsao G, et al. A randomized, double-blind, placebo-controlled trial of ursodeoxycholic acid in primary biliary cirrhosis. *Hepatology* 1995; 22: 759-66.
48. Heathcote EJ, Cauch-Duder K, Walker V, Bailey RJ, Blendis LM, Ghent CM, Michieletti P, et al. The Canadian multicenter double-blind randomized controled trial of ursodeoxycholic acid in primary biliary cirrhosis. *Hepatology* 1994; 19: 1149-56.
49. Lindor KD. Ursodiol for primary sclerosing cholangitis. Mayo Primary Sclerosing Cholangitis-Ursodeoxycholic Acid Study Group. *N Engl J Med* 1997; 336: 691-5.
50. Eriksson LS, Olsson R, Glauman H, Prytz H, Befrits R, Ryden BO, Einarsson K, Lindgren S, Wallerstedt S, Weden M. Ursodeoxycholic acid treatment in patient with primary biliary cirrhosis. A Swedish multicentre, double-blind, randomized controlled study. *Scand J Gastroenterol* 1997; 32: 179-86.
51. Ikeda T, Tozuka S, Noguchi O, Kobayashi F, Sakamoto S, Marumo F, Sato C. Effects of additional administration of colchicine in ursodeoxycholic acid-treated patients with primary biliary cirrhosis: a prospective randomized study. *J Hepatol* 1996; 24: 88-94.
52. Poupon RE, Huet PM, Poupon R, Bonnand AM, Nhieu JT, Zafrani ES. A randomized trial comparing colchicine and ursodeoxycholic acid combination to ursodeoxycholic acid in primary biliary cirrhosis. UDCA-PBC Study Group. *Hepatology* 1996; 24: 1098-103.
53. Leuschner M, Guldutuna S, You T, Hubner K, Bhatti S, Leuschner U. Ursodeoxycholic acid and prednisolone *versus* ursodeoxycholic acid and placebo in the treatment of early stages of primary biliary cirrhosis. *J Hepatol* 1996; 25: 49-57.
54. Wolfhagen FH, van Hoogstraten HJF, van Buuren HR, Van Berge Henegouwen GP, ten Kate FJW, Hop WCJ, van der Hoek EW, Kerbert MJ, van Lijf HH, den Ouden JW, et al. Benefits and risks of 1-year triple therapy with ursodeoxycholic acid, prednisone, and azathioprine in primary biliary cirrhosis: results of a randomized placebo controled trial. Submitted, 1997.
55. Gonzalez-Koch A, Brahm J, Antezana C, Smok G, Cumsile MA. The combination of ursodeoxycholic acid and methotrexate for primary biliary cirrhosis is not better that ursodeoxycholic acid alone. *J Hepatol* 1997; 27: 143-9.
56. Lindor KD, Dickson ER, Jorgensen RA, Anderson ML, Wiesner RH, Gores GJ, Lange SM, Rossi SS, Hofmann AF, Baldus WP. The combination of ursodeoxycholic acid and methotrexate for patients with primary biliary cirrhosis: the results of a pilot study. *Hepatology* 1995; 22: 1158-62.

57. Ricci P, Therneau TM, Malinchoc M, Benson JT, Petz JL, Klintmalm GB, Crippin JS, Wiesner RH, Steers JL, Rakela J, *et al.* A prognostic model for the outcome of liver transplantation in patients with cholestatic liver disease. *Hepatology* 1997; 25: 672-7.
58. Navasa M, Forns X, Sanchez V, Andreu H, Marcos V, Borras JM, Rimola A, Grande L, Garcia Valdecasas JC, Granados A, *et al.* Quality of life, major medical complications and hospital service utilization in patients with primary biliary cirrhosis after liver transplantation. *J Hepatol* 1996; 25: 129-34.
59. Gouw ASH, Haagsma EB, Manns M, Klompmaker IJ, Slooff MJH, Gerber MA. Is there recurrence of primary biliary cirrhosis after liver transplantation? A clinicopathologic study in long-term survivors. *J Hepatol* 1994; 20: 500-7.
60. Knoop M, Bechstein WO, Schrem H, Lobeck H, Hopf U, Neuhaus P. Clinical significance of recurrent primary bilary cirrhosis after liver transplantation. *Transpl Int* 1996; 9 Suppl 1: S115-9.
61. Slapak GI, Saxena R, Portmann B, Gane E, Devlin J, Calne R, Williams R. Graft and systemic disease in long-term survivors of liver transplantation. *Hepatology* 1997; 25: 195-202.
62. Van de Water J, Gerson LB, Ferrell LD, Lake JR, Coppel RL, Batts KP, Wiesner RH, Gershwin ME. Immunohistochemical evidence of disease recurrence after liver transplantation for primary biliary cirrhosis. *Hepatology* 1996; 24: 1079-84.
63. Dimitrewski J, Hubscher SG, Mayer AD, Neuberger JM. Recurrence of primary biliary cirrhosis in the liver allograft: the effect of immunosuppression. *J Hepatol* 1996; 24: 253-7.

Hepatitis C: current concepts

G.M. Dusheiko

Royal Free Hospital and School of Medicine, London, United Kingdom

Summary

Hepatitis C virus (HCV) has a similar organization to pestiviruses and flaviviruses of the family Flaviviridae, but is sufficiently distinct to be classified within its own genus. The total or partial nucleotide sequences obtained from a number of isolates indicate that they may be divided into at least six major types with component subtypes based upon nucleotide homology. Infection with hepatitis C is most clearly seen after transfusion of whole-blood products, but in many countries the disease has been acquired by community acquired transmission. There is a high prevalence of hepatitis C in past or current intravenous drug abusers, haemophiliacs, thalassaemics, haemodialyzed patients and transplant recipients. The pathogenesis of the disease is poorly understood. A $CD4^+$ proliferative T-lymphocyte response to recombinant viral antigens has been found in infected individuals with different clinical courses. Immunity to HCV is not readily elicited. Repeated episodes of hepatitis may be due to the emergence of mutants of HCV not neutralized by circulating antibody. The acute disease may occasionally resolve completely with clearance of HCV RNA from serum. A suitable immunodiagnostic test for resolved infection and immunity is not available. The majority of chronic cases will not have been preceded by an episode of clinically apparent, icteric hepatitis. Fifty to seventy-five percent of patients with type C post-transfusion or sporadic hepatitis continue to have abnormal serum aminotransferases after 12 months, and chronic hepatitis histologically.
Cirrhosis develops in approximately 10-20% of patients with chronic disease within 10 years. It is not easy to project the prognosis for patients seen at one point in time. Episodes of hepatic necrosis may progress at variable rates to cirrhosis. Ideally HCV RNA should be measured in all patients to confirm viraemia, but the test is not generally available for routine diagnosis. Individuals with chronic hepatitis C with elevated ALT and chronic hepatitis histologically should be considered for antiviral therapy. Unfortunately responsiveness to alpha interferon remains somewhat unpredictable; factors which predict a greater likelihood of response are now being studied. Studies of ribavirin and

alpha interferon used together indicate that relapse rates are reduced, and up to 35% of relapsed patients may have a sustained virological response rate after treatment for six months with alpha interferon and ribavirin.

Virology

The complete nucleotide sequence of the HCV genome has been determined in a number of isolates and shown to be a positive RNA of approximately 9,400 nucleotides. This consists of one long open reading frame encoding a polyprotein of 3,010-3,033 amino acids which is cleaved into functionally distinct polypeptides during or after translation. The virus has similar organization to pestiviruses and flaviviruses of the family Flaviviridae, but is sufficiently distinct to be classified within its own genus. The nucleocapsid and envelope proteins are encoded at the 5' end of the genome, while the non-structural elements are downstream of this *(figure 1)*. The total or partial nucleotide sequences obtained from a number of isolates indicate that they may be divided into at least six major types with component subtypes based upon nucleotide homology [1-4].

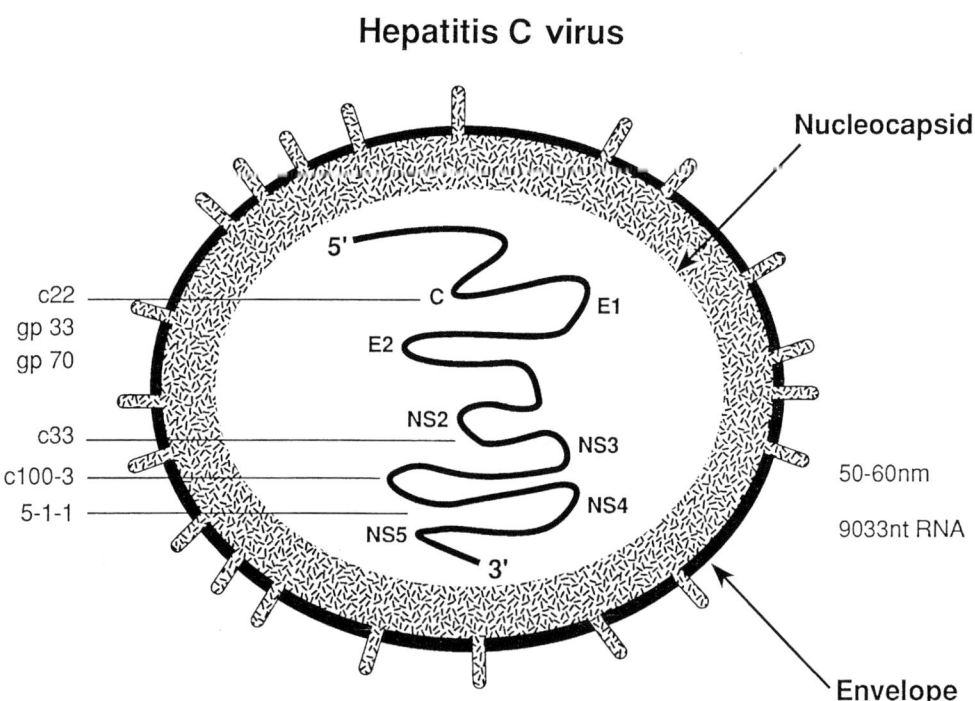

Figure 1. Putative structure of the hepatitis C virus particle. Expressed proteins are used as antigens in enzyme linked immunoassays to detect diagnostic antibodies in serum.

There are hypervariable regions especially in the E1 and E2 domains. These regions, especially those of the envelope glycoproteins, may be important antigenic sites and their variability may be critical to persistence of infection and immunopathogenesis.

Transmission and epidemiology

Infection with hepatitis C is most clearly seen after transfusion of whole-blood products, but in many countries the disease has been acquired by community acquired transmission. There is a high prevalence of hepatitis C in haemophiliacs, thalassaemics, haemodialyzed patients, transplant recipients, intravenous drug abusers, and in some countries, dentists. Intrafamilial transmission may occur, but appears to be relatively infrequent in developed countries. Maternal infant transmission has been documented in mothers with higher levels of viraemia, but also appears to be infrequent [5].

Pathogenesis

The pathogenic mechanisms that result in hepatitis are unknown. Lymphocytes are typically observed within the hepatic parenchyma, but the functional characteristics of these cells have not been fully defined. However in the liver $CD8^+$ cell subsets predominate over $CD4^+$ subsets in patients with chronic hepatitis C [6]. The mechanism of hepatitis in acute hepatitis C has not been well studied. T cell clones reactive with non-A, non-B infected hepatocytes from patients with chronic hepatitis have been identified [7]. Liver-infiltrating lymphocytes from subjects with chronic HCV hepatitis have been cloned at limiting dilution and tested for HCV-specific cytolytic activity using autologous target cells infected with vaccinia viruses expressing recombinant HCV antigens or sensitized with synthetic HCV peptides. HCV- specific HLA class I-restricted CTL were identified that recognized epitopes in variable regions of either the envelope or nonstructural proteins. Thus HCV-specific CTL can be demonstrated at the site of tissue damage in persons with chronic HCV hepatitis, which may have a pathogenic role [8].

A $CD4^+$ proliferative T-lymphocyte response to recombinant viral antigens has been found in infected individuals with different clinical courses. All viral proteins were immunogenic for T cells, although NS4 was the most immunogenic. There may be a correlation between the presence of $CD4^+$ T cell responses to core and a benign course of infection in viraemic carriers with minimal hepatitis [9].

Immunity to HCV is not readily elicited [10]. These episodes of hepatitis may be due to the emergence of mutants of HCV not neutralized by circulating antibody. However this hypothesis has to be proven by careful assessment of nucleotide sequence change in patients with hepatitis C, and corresponding antibody reactivity to viral epitopes. There can be an overlap between hepatitis C infection and autoimmune hepatitis. The humoral response to a host cellular gene-derived epitope GOR (anti-GOR) has been reported to be associated with chronic HCV infection [11, 12]. Anti-Gor has been found in high proportion of anti-LKM1 antibody positive patients with anti-HCV, but not in anti-LKM positive patients negative for anti-HCV (type IIb vs IIa autoimmune chronic hepatitis) [13]. Immune cross reaction of P450IID6 epitopes and hepatitis C proteins may explain the occurrence of anti-LKM antibodies in patients [14].

Clinical and laboratory features

Acute HCV infection

The mean incubation period of HCV is 6-12 weeks. However, with large inocula, such as following administration of factor VIII, the incubation period is reduced [15, 16]. The acute course of HCV infection is clinically mild, and the peak serum ALT elevations are less than those encountered in acute hepatitis A or B. Only 25% of cases are icteric. During the early clinical phase the serum ALT levels may fluctuate, and may become normal or near normal, making the determination of true convalescence difficult *(figure 2)*.

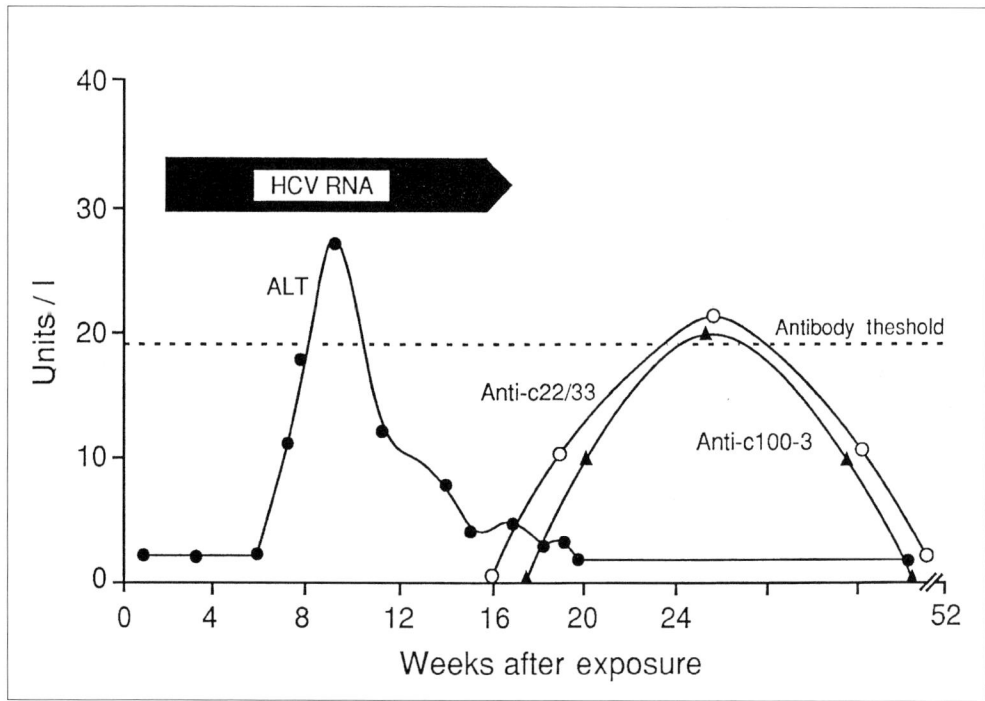

Figure 2. Serological course in acute resolving hepatitis C.

The average time from transfusion to seroconversion is of the order of 7-8 weeks with the second generation tests: anti-c33 or anti-c22 not infrequently appear a week or two earlier than anti-c100-3. Seroconversion occurs much less frequently, and in lower titre, in acute self-limiting infections compared with those that progress to become chronic [17, 18]. Serological testing now indicates that seroconversion to anti-HCV occurs in 85-100% of patients with chronic post-transfusion NANB hepatitis [19]. A proportion of patients with post-transfusion and sporadically acquired NANB patients remain anti-HCV seronegative however.

The acute disease may resolve completely with clearance of HCV RNA from serum. A suitable immunodiagnostic test for resolved infection and immunity is not available.

Serum HCV RNA has been detected within one to three weeks of transfusion in patients with hepatitis C, and usually lasts less than 4 months in patients with acute self-limited hepatitis C, but may persist for decades in patients with chronic disease [20, 21].

Chronic hepatitis C

The majority of cases will not have been preceded by an episode of clinically apparent, icteric hepatitis. Fifty to seventy-five percent of patients with type C post-transfusion or sporadic hepatitis continue to have abnormal serum aminotransferase levels after 12 months, and chronic hepatitis histologically [22]. Serum aminotransferases decline from the peak values encountered in the acute phase of the disease, but typically remain 2-8 fold abnormal. The serum ALT concentrations may fluctuate over time, and may even intermittently be normal *(figure 3)*.

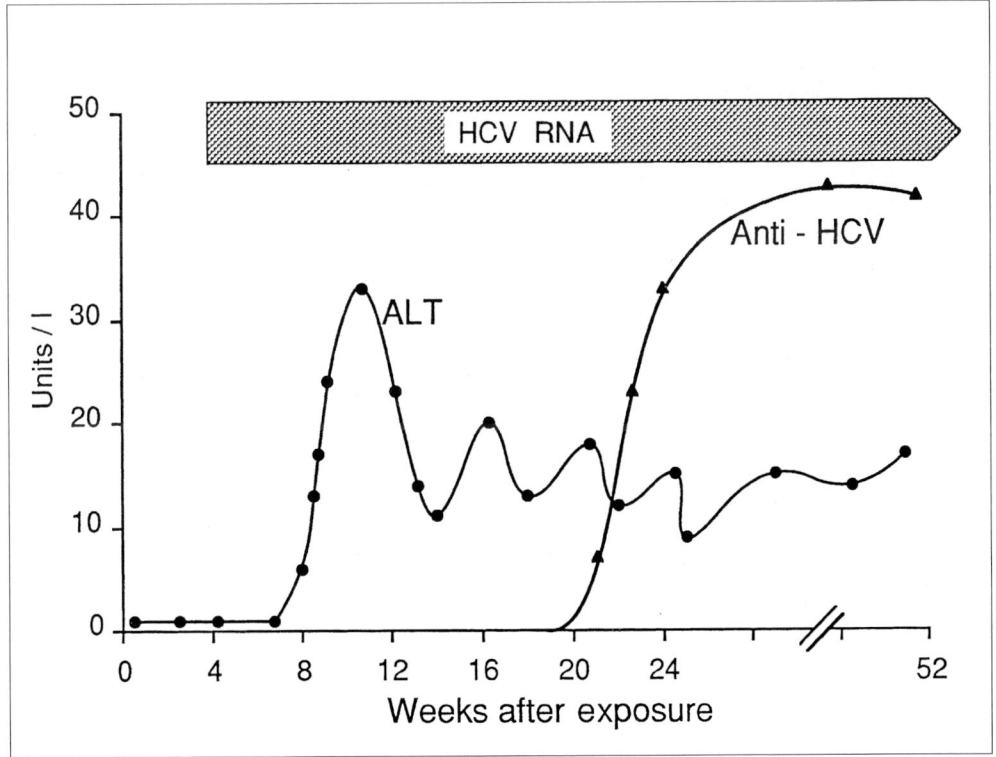

Figure 3. Serological course in acute hepatitis C progressing to chronic disease.

Many patients have a sustained elevation of the serum aminotransferases. Cirrhosis develops in approximately 10-20% of patients with chronic disease within 10 years, albeit that the cirrhosis remains indolent and only slowly progressive for a prolonged period [21, 23-25]. The disease is not necessarily benign however, and rapidly progressive cirrhosis can occur. Older age at infection, concomitant alcohol abuse, concurrent HBV or HIV infection or other illness may be important aggravating co-factors. Older patients may present with complications of cirrhosis, or even HCC. With progressive disease, the laboratory values become progressively more abnormal. The finding of AST greater than ALT, low albumin and prolonged prothrombin time suggest cirrhosis. Low levels of autoantibodies may also become detectable.

Anti-HCV persists for years and even decades in chronic hepatitis C but may decline in titre or disappear with resolution. A small percentage of patients appear to permanently eradicate HCV RNA after chronic infection but this usually less than 10% [17, 26].

HCV RNA usually persists in patients with abnormal serum aminotransferases and anti-HCV. Although most patients with raised serum ALT are HCV RNA positive, the converse is not always true. Isolates of HCV in individual patients may show nucleotide substitutions with time, suggesting that the HCV RNA mutates at a rate similar to those of other RNA viruses [27]. The emergence of a mutant population does not always correlate with peaks in ALT.

It is not easy to project the prognosis for patients seen at one point in time. Episodes of hepatic necrosis may progress at variable rates to cirrhosis and conversely the lesion may revert in some patients to inactive hepatitis. Cirrhosis may develop in patients with an initial mild histological pattern; the mechanism for this transition is not known but may occur after repeated attacks of lobular necrosis associated with piecemeal necrosis. A relationship between histological exacerbations and an episodic clinical course is not proven however. The morphological features of cirrhosis due to HCV are not specific to the disease; in the earlier stages, lymphoid aggregates may be seen.

The infection causes systemic disease, and may be associated with a number of systemic complications including a form of autoimmune hepatitis, cryoglobulinaemia [28], porphyria cutanea tarda, lymphocytic sialedinitis, and membranous glomerulonephritis.

Diagnosis

Expressed proteins of this virus protein are now used as antigens in enzyme-linked immunoassays to detect diagnostic antibodies in serum [29]. To date it has not been possible to detect viral antigens routinely. Thus the detection of antibodies to HCV has become important as an indication of past or present infection. The second and third generation antibody assays incorporate extra HCV derived recombinant proteins, which improve the sensitivity of the assay [30, 31]. Antibodies to c22c are an earlier finding and occur more frequently than those to c100-3, during the course of HCV infection. This is probably due to conservation of amino acid sequence in this region, together with greater immunogenicity of the core peptide. A protein derived from the NS3 and NS4 regions (c200) or a smaller fragment of it (c33c) from NS3 alone, is also included in the second generation assays. These antibodies are probably not neutralizing, in that they are found throughout chronic infection. The third generation of antibody assays also incorporate epitopes derived from the NS5 region. Antibodies to envelope proteins have been detected in viraemic patients, and it is therefore uncertain whether such antibodies are neutralizing [32-35]. IgM responses to HCV c100-3 antigen have been investigated in acute and chronic disease [36].

Supplemental tests for antibody to HCV

The most widely used method is the recombinant immunoblot assay (RIBA) (Chiron Corporation) in which antibodies are sought to recombinant antigens of HCV coated on nitrocellulose strips. Samples are regarded as confirmed positive if antibodies to two or more of the HCV proteins are present and indeterminate if only antibody to one antigen is found. The value of RIBA in excluding false positive results has been extensively demonstrated, as has correlation between RIBA positivity and viraemia [37, 38].

Detection of viral genome

Direct detection of HCV RNA by conventional nucleic acid hybridisation techniques is difficult, but HCV RNA can be detected by an amplification technique (PCR) [39, 40]. Using this method, HCV RNA can be detected in majority of anti-HCV positive patients. The selection of PCR primers from the 5' region results in a great improvement in the sensitivity of the assay [41, 42]. Sample handling can affect sensitivity. Methods for quantification have until now been based on dilution analysis. More accurate methods of HCV RNA quantification are being developed for clinical use and measuring response to antiviral therapy [43, 44]. The sequencing of PCR products enables information on genome diversity between isolates to be gathered. This will be important if, as has been suggested, the clinical outcome and response to treatment are determined by the infecting subtype [45].

Treatment

Acute HCV infection

The management of acute sporadic or transfusion related HCV infection includes conventional supportive treatment and specific antiviral therapy. The disease may be relatively silent in the acute phase, as most (75%) patients are not jaundiced, and have only non-specific symptoms. Current tests should enable a diagnosis to be made in many if the disease is suspected. The diagnosis may require testing for HCV RNA, as some patients may not have anti-HCV at the time that serum aminotransferases are elevated. Anti-HCV may be detectable particularly in severe, icteric cases, and in most of those patients destined to go on to chronic disease. Antibody can be detected earlier by third generation antibody tests.

Recent phase II trials with alpha and beta interferon, which have included 8 weeks to 12 months of therapy and higher doses (up to 6 mu), have provided more convincing evidence that risk of chronic hepatitis can be reduced. However, it is not always clear whether treatment has benefited those patients who might have been convalescing spontaneously, and whether late relapses will still occur in those patients who remain HCV RNA positive. However, if a diagnosis of acute hepatitis C can be made, and the patient does not appear to be convalescing 2-4 months after the onset of the disease, alpha interferon can be considered at a dose of 3-6 mu three times weekly for at least 4 to 6 months.

Chronic HCV infection

Ideally HCV RNA should be measured in all patients to confirm viraemia, but the test is not generally available for routine diagnosis. If the test is reproducibly positive, then serum aminotransferases, bilirubin, alkaline phosphatase, and prothrombin time should be measured in referred blood donors. In patients whose lifestyle or geographic origin suggest that they are at risk of other forms of viral hepatitis, HBsAg and HIV infection need also be considered. Because autoimmune hepatitis is treated differently, it is particularly advisable to exclude this diagnosis by measuring the titres of anti-smooth muscle, and anti-liver kidney microsomal antibodies even in those with a positive anti-HCV test, and to measure HCV RNA in anti-HCV positive patients in whom interferon is contemplated.

Individuals with chronic hepatitis C with elevated ALT and chronic hepatitis histologically should be considered for antiviral therapy. Large placebo controlled studies have indicated that approximately 50% of patients will have normal serum aminotransferases at the end of treatment courses of alpha interferon of approximately 3 million units three times a week for six months [46, 47].

Serum HCV RNA may become undetectable in patients after 4-8 weeks of alpha interferon treatment in patients who respond, but an undetectable HCV RNA at the end of treatment does not preclude relapse in patients.

However, six months after stopping treatment, one half of the responsive patients will promptly relapse. Serum aminotransferases usually increase in patients who are HCV RNA positive at the end of therapy, although in some cases the relapse may be delayed for several months [48]. Fifteen to 20% of patients have a prolonged response to therapy and do not again develop elevated serum aminotransferases [49]. These patients also remain negative for HCV RNA.

There is most information about 3 mu three times weekly given for six months. It is clear that treatment for 12 months improves the response rate. Other regimens are being evaluated, and there is a suggestion that higher doses may be beneficial [50]. Initiating therapy with a somewhat higher dose of 15-18 mu per week, and prolonging therapy for a year may result in lower relapse rates; however, higher doses are associated with greater toxicity. Treatment should not be continued beyond three months in patients who do not have reduced levels of serum ALT. Responsive patients usually exhibit histological improvement, and may have a decrease in collagen III propeptide concentrations [51].

Unfortunately responsiveness to alpha interferon remains somewhat unpredictable; factors which predict a greater likelihood of response are now being studied. Multivariate analysis of several pre-treatment parameters indicate that patients without cirrhosis are more responsive to interferon, and are more likely to have a sustained response. The influence of genotypes of hepatitis C is the subject of considerable interest at present, as is the association between lower levels of viraemia and response. In large controlled trials it has become apparent that genotype type 1b, and 1a are associated with a relatively poor response to interferon therapy [52-54]. Patients with diverse circulating quasispecies may be less responsive to therapy than those with a single major species *(figure 4)*. Improved responses have been observed in patients with lower levels of circulating HCV RNA [55]. Unfortunately, the issue remains complex: there is not yet a standardised system for quantitating concentrations of HCV RNA in serum and genotyping and HCV RNA quantitation are not generally available to clinicians. However, when serotyping becomes available together with quantitation of HCV RNA, clinicians may be able to rationalize the use of interferon, and the dose required.

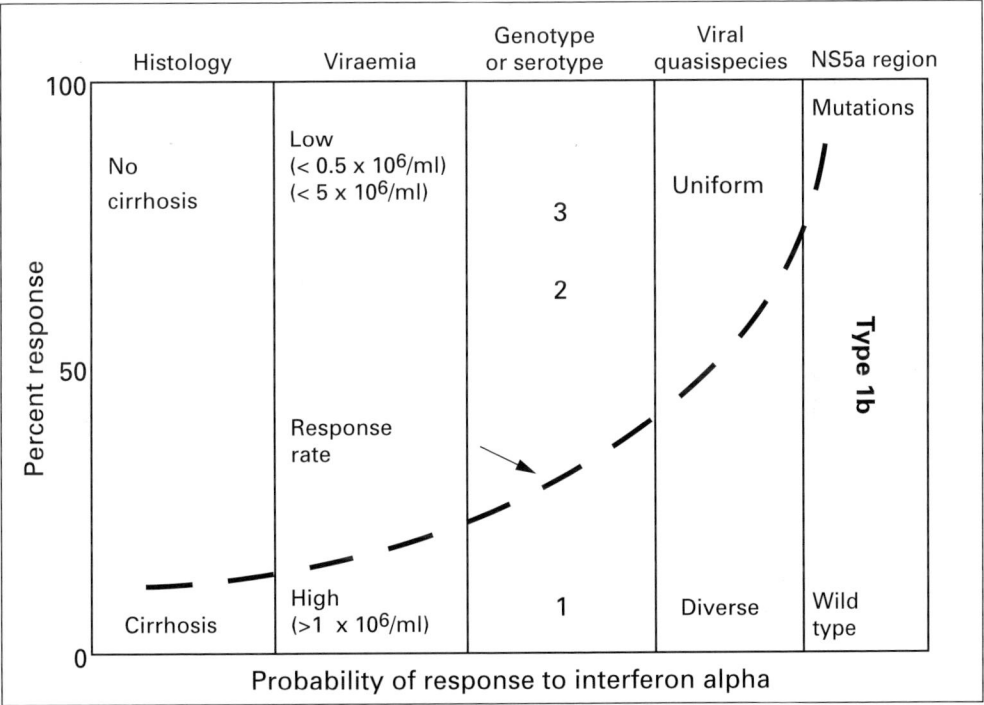

Figure 4. Chart showing factors which determine the probability of responsiveness to a six, and possibly twelve months course of alpha interferon for chronic hepatitis C.

It is reasonable to infer that those patients with normal serum ALT a year after stopping interferon treatment, and negative for HCV RNA a year after stopping therapy, with histologically improved disease activity have had a good response. HCV antigens may be cleared from the liver with successful treatment [56].

Some patients may actually worsen on treatment with interferon, and develop increased serum aminotransferases. A positive anti-HCV antibody in patients with autoimmune disease remains a pitfall in diagnosis, which has implications for treatment. Such patients require confirmation by HCV RNA, as they may optimally require corticosteroid therapy rather than alpha interferon [57]. It is possible that such patients have an underlying autoimmune status associated with hepatitis C and exacerbated by interferon treatment. For such patients, and for patients who do not respond to treatment, ribavirin may be an alternative [58].

Ribavirin and interferon

Ribavirin is a synthetic guanosine nucleotide analogue, which possesses a broad spectrum of activity against both DNA and RNA viruses *in vitro* and *in vivo* [59]. The drug exerts its action after intracellular phosphorylation to mono, di- and triphosphate nucleotides. The precise mode of action probably includes direct inhibition of the viral mRNA polymerase complex, and possibly enhancement of macrophage inhibition of viral replication.

The pharmacokinetics of ribavirin have been studied. The bioavailability of oral formulations has been calculated at 19-65% (compared with IV administration). The distribution half life is 1-3 hours, but the terminal half life is prolonged (27-52 hours) perhaps due to sequestration within red cells and other tissues. Ribavirin is concentrated 10-50 fold in red blood cells, and crosses the blood brain barrier. Peak plasma levels range from 5-13 uM after single oral doses of 600-2,400 mg. The excretion of the drug is predominantly renal.

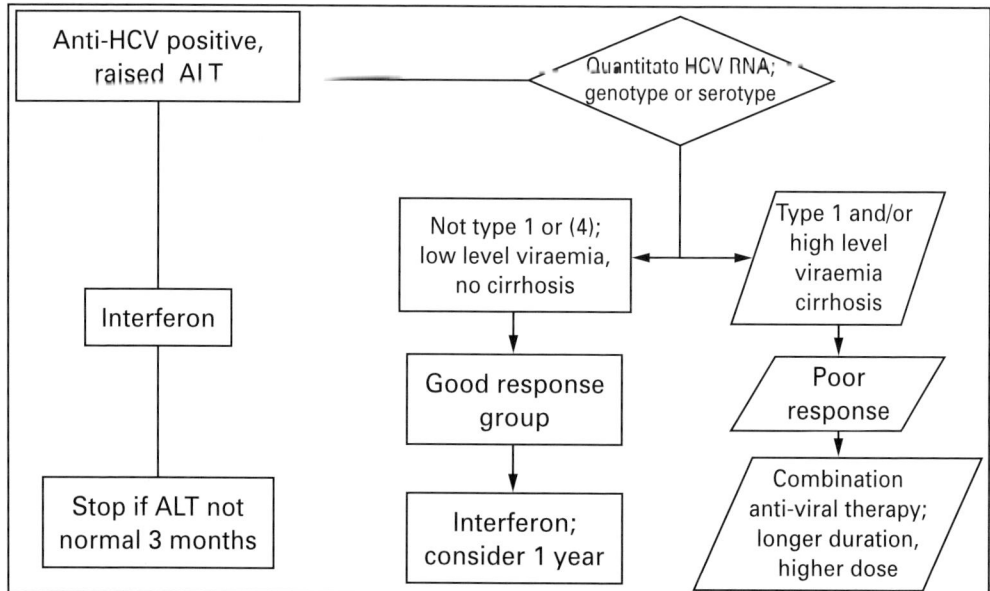

Figure 5. Approach to the treatment of chronic hepatitis C. Some physicians may prefer to treat all patients to determine the response to alpha interferon used alone. It may be possible however to distinguish likely poor responders who are better treated with a combination of antiviral agents.

The major side effects of the drug that have been reported include anaemia, a metallic taste, dry mouth, flatulence, dyspepsia, nausea, headaches, irritability, emotional lability, fatigue, insomnia, skin rashes and myalgia. Mild reversible anaemia is common. Modest increases in uric acid have been reported.

Studies of ribavirin and alpha interferon used together indicate that relapse rates are reduced, and up to 35% of relapsed patients may have a sustained virological response rate after treatment for six months with alpha interferon and ribavirin. It may be possible to distinguish patients who are better treated with a combination of antiviral agents *(figure 5)*.

Vaccination

There are no vaccines for the prevention of hepatitis C. Viral heterogeneity is likely to make the development of vaccine a difficult task. Perhaps DNA vaccination will offer the most suitable strategy [60, 61].

References

1. Chan SW, Simmonds P, McOmish F, Yap PL, Mitchell R, Dow B, Follett E. Serological responses to infection with three different types of hepatitis C virus. *Lancet* 1991; 338: 1391.
2. Simmonds P, McOmish F, Yap PL, Chan SW, Lin CK, Dusheiko G, Saeed AA, Holmes EC. Sequence variability in the 5' non-coding region of hepatitis C virus: identification of a new virus type and restrictions on sequence diversity. *J Gen Virol* 1993; 74: 661-8.
3. Simmonds P, Holmes EC, Cha TA, Chan SW, McOmish F, Irvine B, Beall E, Yap PL, Kolberg J, Urdea MS. Classification of hepatitis C virus into six major genotypes and a series of subtypes by phylogenetic analysis of the NS-5 region. *J Gen Virol* 1993; 74: 2391-9.
4. McOmish F, Chan SW, Dow BC, Gillon J, Frame WD, Crawford RJ, Yap PL, Follett EAC, Simmonds P. Detection of three types of hepatitis C virus in blood donors: investigation of type-specific differences in serologic reactivity and rate of alanine aminotransferase abnormalities. *Transfusion* 1993; 33: 7-13.
5. Thaler MM, Park CK, Landers DV, Wara DW, Houghton M, Veereman-Wauters G, Sweet RL, Han JH. Vertical transmission of hepatitis C virus. *Lancet* 1991; 338: 17-8.
6. Onji M, Kikuchi T, Kumon I, Masumoto T, Nadano S, Kajino K, Horiike N, Ohta Y. Intrahepatic lymphocyte subpopulations and HLA class I antigen expression by hepatocytes in chronic hepatitis C. *Hepato-Gastroenterol* 1992; 39: 340-3.
7. Imawari M, Nomura M, Kaieda T, Moriyama T, Oshimi K, Nakamura I, Gunji T, Ohnishi S, Ishikawa T, Nakagama H, et al. Establishment of a human T-cell clone cytotoxic for both autologous and allogeneic hepatocytes from chronic hepatitis patients with type non-A, non-B virus. *Proc Natl Acad Sci USA* 1989; 86: 2883-7.
8. Koziel MJ, Dudley D, Wong JT, Dienstag J, Houghton M, Ralston R, Walker BD. Intrahepatic cytotoxic T lymphocytes specific for hepatitis C virus in persons with chronic hepatitis. *J Immunol* 1992; 149: 3339-44.
9. Botarelli P, Brunetto MR, Minutello MA, Calvo P, Unutmaz D, Weiner AJ, Choo QL, Shuster JR, Kuo G, Bonino F, et al. T-lymphocyte response to hepatitis C virus in different clinical courses of infection. *Gastroenterology* 1993; 104: 580-7.

10. Farci P, Alter HJ, Govindarajan S, Wong DC, Engle R, Lesniewski RR, Mushahwar IK, Desai SM, Miller RH, Ogata N, Purcell RH. Lack of protective immunity against reinfection with hepatitis C virus. *Science* 1992; 258: 135-40.
11. Mishiro S, Hoshi Y, Takeda K, Yoshikawa A, Gotanda T, Takahashi K, Akahane Y, Yoshizawa H, Okamoto H, Tsuda F, *et al*. Non-A, non-B hepatitis specific antibodies directed at host-derived epitope: implication for an autoimmune process. *Lancet* 1990; 336: 1400-3.
12. Mehta SU, Mishiro S, Sekiguchi K, Leung T, Dawson GJ, Pendy LM, Peterson DA, Devare SG. Immune response to GOR, a marker for non-A, non-B hepatitis and its correlation with hepatitis C virus infection. *J Clin Immunol* 1992; 12: 178-84.
13. Michel G, Ritter A, Gerken G, Meyer zum Buschenfelde KH, Decker R. Anti-GOR and hepatitis C virus in autoimmune liver diseases [see comments]. *Lancet* 1992; 339: 267-9.
14. Manns MP, Griffin KJ, Sullivan KF, Johnson EF. LKM-1 autoantibodies recognize a short linear sequence in P450IID6, a cytochrome P-450 monooxygenase. *J Clin Invest* 1991; 88: 1370-8.
15. Bamber M, Murray A, Arborgh BAM, *et al*. Short incubation non-A, non-B hepatitis transmitted by factor VIII concentrates in patients with congenital coagulation disorders. *Gut* 1981; 22: 854-9.
16. Lim SG, Lee CA, Charman H, Tilsed G, Griffiths PD, Kernoff PBA. Hepatitis C antibody assay in a longitudinal study of haemophiliacs. *Br J Haematol* 1991; 78: 398-402.
17. Alter HJ, Purcell RH, Shih JW, Melpolder JC, Houghton M, Choo Q, Kuo G. Detection of antibody to hepatitis C virus in prospectively followed transfusion recipients with acute and chronic non-A, non-B hepatitis. *N Engl J Med* 1989; 321: 1494-500.
18. Nishioka K, Watanabe J, Furuta S, Tanaka E, Suzuki H, Iino S, Tsuji T, Yano M, Kuo G, Choo QL, *et al*. Antibody to the hepatitis C virus in acute hepatitis and chronic liver diseases in Japan. *Liver* 1991; 11: 65-70.
19. Esteban JI, Gonzalez A, Hernandez JM, Viladomiu L, Sanchez C, Lopez-Talavera JC, Lucea D, Martin-Vega C, Vidal X, Esteban R, *et al*. Evaluation of antibodies to hepatitis C virus in a study of transfusion-associated hepatitis. *N Engl J Med* 1990; 323: 1107-12.
20. Farci P, Alter HJ, Wong D, Miller RH, Shih JW, Jett B, Purcell RH. A long-term study of hepatitis C virus replication in non-A, non-B hepatitis. *N Engl J Med* 1991; 325: 98-104.
21. Patel A, Sherlock S, Dusheiko G, Scheuer PJ, Ellis LA, Ashratzadeh P. Clinical course and histological correlations in post-transfusion hepatitis C: the Royal Free Hospital experience. *Eur J Gastroenterol Hepatol* 1991; 3: 491-5.
22. Lee SD, Hwang SJ, Lu RH, Lai KH, Tsai YT, Lo KJ. Antibodies to hepatitis C virus in prospectively followed patients with posttransfusion hepatitis. *J Infect Dis* 1991; 163: 1354-7.
23. Berman M, Alter HJ, Ishak KG, Purcell RH, Jones EA. The chronic sequelae of non-A, non-B hepatitis. *Ann Intern Med* 1979; 91: 1-6.
24. Koretz RL, Stone O, Gitnick GL. The long term course of non-A, non-B post-transfusion hepatitis. *Gastroenterology* 1980; 79: 893-8.
25. Mattsson L, Weiland O, Glaumann H. Chronic non-A, non-B hepatitis developed after transfusions, illicit self-injections or sporadically. Outcome during long-term follow-up-a comparison. *Liver* 1989; 9: 120-7.
26. Tanaka E, Kiyosawa K, Sodeyama T, Nakano Y, Yoshizawa K, Hayata T, Shimizu S, Nakatsuji Y, Koike Y, Furuta S. Significance of antibody to hepatitis C virus in Japanese patients with viral hepatitis: relationship between anti-HCV antibody and the prognosis of non-A, non-B post-transfusion hepatitis. *J Med Virol* 1991; 33: 117-22.
27. Ogata N, Alter HJ, Miller RH, Purcell RH. Nucleotide sequence and mutation rate of the H strain of hepatitis C virus. *Proc Natl Acad Sci USA* 1991; 88: 3392-6.
28. Dammacco F, Sansonno D. Antibodies to hepatitis C virus in essential mixed cryoglobulinaemia [see comments]. *Clin Exp Immunol* 1992; 87: 352-6.
29. Choo QL, Weiner AJ, Overby LR, Kuo G, Houghton M, Bradley DW. Hepatitis C virus: the major causative agent of viral non-A, non-B hepatitis. *Br Med Bull* 1990; 46: 423-41.

30. Aach RD, Stevens CE, Hollinger BF, Mosley JW, Peterson DA, Taylor P, Johnson RG, Barbosa LH, Nemo GJ. Hepatitis C virus infection in post-transfusion hepatitis. An analysis with first and second-generation assays. *N Engl J Med* 1991; 325: 1325-9.
31. McHutchison JG, Person JL, Govindarajan S, Valinluck B, Gore T, Lee SR, Nelles M, Polito A, Chien D, Dinello R, Quan S, Kuo G, Redeker AG. Improved detection of hepatitis C virus antibodies in high-risk populations. *Hepatology* 1992; 15: 19-25.
32. Schlesinger JJ, Brandriss MW, Cropp CB, Monath TP. Protection against yellow fever in monkeys by immunization with yellow fever virus nonstructural protein NS1. *J Virol* 1986; 60: 1153-5.
33. Donis RO, Corapi W, Dubovi EJ. Neutralizing monoclonal antibodies to bovine viral diarrhoea virus bind to the 56K to 58K glycoprotein. *J Gen Virol* 1988; 69: 77-86.
34. Weiland E, Stark R, Haas B, Rumenapf T, Meyers G, Thiel HJ. Pestivirus glycoprotein which induces neutralizing antibodies forms part of a disulfide-linked heterodimer. *J Virol* 1990; 64: 3563-9.
35. Van-Zijl M, Wensvoort G, de Kluyver E, Hulst M, van der Gulden H, Gielkens A, Berns A, Moormann R. Live attenuated pseudorabies virus expressing envelope glycoprotein E1 of hog cholera virus protects swine against both pseudorabies and hog cholera. *J Virol* 1991; 65: 2761-5.
36. Chen PJ, Wang JT, Hwang LH, Yang YH, Hsieh CL, Kao JH, Sheu JC, Lai MY, Wang TH, Chen DS. Transient immunoglobulin M antibody response to hepatitis C virus capsid antigen in posttransfusion hepatitis C: putative serological marker for acute viral infection. *Proc Natl Acad Sci USA* 1992; 89: 5971-5.
37. Ebeling F, Naukkarinen R, Leikola J. Recombinant immunoblot assay for hepatitis C virus antibody as predictor of infectivity [letter]. *Lancet* 1990; 335: 982-3.
38. Stillwagon GB, Order SE, Guse C, Leibel SA, Asbell SO, Klein JL, Leichner PK. Prognostic factors in unresectable hepatocellular cancer: Radiation Therapy Oncology Group Study 83-01. *Int J Radiat Oncol Biol Phys* 1991; 20: 65-71.
39. Weiner AJ, Kuo G, Bradley DW, Bonino F, Saracco G, Lee C, Rosenblatt J, Choo Q, Houghton M. Detection of hepatitis C viral sequences in non-A, non-B hepatitis. *Lancet* 1990; 335: 13.
40. Kato N, Yokosuka O, Omata M, Hosoda K, Ohto M. Detection of hepatitis C virus ribonucleic acid in the serum by amplification with polymerase chain reaction. *J Clin Invest* 1990; 86: 1764-7.
41. Garson JA, Ring C, Tuke P, Tedder RS. Enhanced detection by PCR of hepatitis C virus RNA [letter]. *Lancet* 1990; 336: 878-9.
42. Okamoto H, Okada S, Sugiyama Y, Tanaka T, Sugai Y, Akahane Y, Machida A, Mishiro S, Yoshizawa H, Miyakawa Y, *et al.* Detection of hepatitis C virus RNA by a two-stage polymerase chain reaction with two pairs of primers deduced from the 5'-noncoding region. *Jpn J Exp Med* 1990; 60: 215-22.
43. Kato N, Hijikata M, Nakagawa M, Ootsuyama Y, Muraiso K, Ohkoshi S, Shimotohno K. Molecular structure of the Japanese hepatitis C viral genome. *FEBS Lett* 1991; 280: 325-8.
44. Chung RT, Dienstag JL, Kaplan LM. Precise quantitation of hepatitis C RNA using a competitive polymerase chain reaction: correlation of clinical course with levels of circulating RNA. *Hepatology* 1991; 14: 65A.
45. Takada N, Takase S, Enomoto N, Takada A, Date T. Clinical backgrounds of the patients having different types of hepatitis C virus genomes. *J Hepatol* 1992; 14: 35-40.
46. Davis GL, Balart LA, Schiff ER, Lindsay K, Bodenheimer HCJ, Perrillo RP, Carey W, Jacobson IM, Payne J, Dienstag JL, *et al.* Treatment of chronic hepatitis C with recombinant interferon alfa. A multicenter randomized, controlled trial. *N Engl J Med* 1989; 321: 1501-6.
47. Di Bisceglie AM, Martin P, Kassianides C, Lisker-Melman M, Murray L, Waggoner J, Goodman Z, Banks SM, Hoofnagle JH. Recombinant interferon alfa therapy for chronic hepatitis C. A randomized, double-blind, placebo-controlled trial. *N Engl J Med* 1989; 321: 1506-10.
48. Chayama K, Saitoh S, Arase Y, Ikeda K, Matsumoto T, Sakai Y, Kobayashi M, Unakami M, Morinaga T, Kumada H. Effect of interferon administration on serum hepatitis C virus RNA in patients with chronic hepatitis C. *Hepatology* 1991; 13: 1040-3.

49. Varagona G, Brown D, Kibbler H, Scheuer P, Ashrafzadeh P, Sherlock S, McIntyre N, Dusheiko G. Response, relapse and retreatment rates and viraemia in chronic hepatitis C treated with α2b interferon. A phase III study. *Eur J Gastroent Hepatol* 1992; 4: 707-12.
50. Kakumu S, Arao M, Yoshioka K, Hayashi H, Kusakabe A, Hirofuji H, Kawabe M. Recombinant human alpha-interferon therapy for chronic non-A, non-B hepatitis: second report. *Am J Gastroenterol* 1990; 85: 655-9.
51. Schvarcz R, Glaumann H, Weiland O, Norkrans G, Wejstal R, Fryden A. Histological outcome in interferon α-2b treated patients with chronic posttransfusion non-A, non-B hepatitis. *Liver* 1991; 11: 30-8.
52. Okamoto H, Sugiyama Y, Okada S, Kurai K, Akahane Y, Sugai Y, Tanaka T, Sato K, Tsuda F, Miyakawa Y, Mayumi M. Typing hepatitis C virus by polymerase chain reaction with type-specific primers: application to clinical surveys and tracing infectious sources. *J Gen Virol* 1992; 73: 673-9.
53. Kanai K, Kako M, Okamoto H. HCV genotypes in chronic hepatitis C and response to interferon. *Lancet* 1992; 339: 1543.
54. Okamoto H, Kanai N, Mishiro S. Full-length nucleotide sequence of a Japanese hepatitis C virus isolate (HC-J1) with high homology to USA isolates. *Nucleic Acids Res* 1992; 20: 6410.
55. Yamada G, Takahashi M, Tsuji T, Yoshizawa H, Okamoto H. Quantitative HCV RNA and effect of interferon therapy in chronic hepatitis C. *Dig Dis Sci* 1992; 37: 1926-7.
56. Krawczynski K, Beach MJ, Bradley DW, Kuo G, Di Bisceglie AM, Houghton M, Reyes GR, Kim JP, Choo QL, Alter MJ. Hepatitis C virus antigen in hepatocytes: immunomorphologic detection and identification. *Gastroenterology* 1992; 103: 622-9.
57. Czaja AJ, Taswell HF, Rakela J, Schimek CM. Frequency and significance of antibody to hepatitis C virus in severe corticosteroid-treated autoimmune chronic active hepatitis [see comments]. *Mayo Clin Proc* 1991; 66: 572-82.
58. Reichard O, Andersson J, Schvarcz R, Weiland O. Ribavirin treatment for chronic hepatitis C. *Lancet* 1991; 337: 1058-61.
59. Fernandez H, Banks G, Smith R. Ribavirin: a clinical overview. *Eur J Epidemiol* 1986; 2: 1-14.
60. Tedeschi V, Akatsuka T, Shih JWK, Battegay M, Feinstone SM. A specific antibody response to HCV E2 elicited in mice by intramuscular inoculation of plasmid DNA containing coding sequences for E2. *Hepatology* 1997; 25: 459-62.
61. Saito T, Sherman GJ, Kurokohchi K, Guo ZP, Donets M, Yu MYW, Berzofsky JA, Akatsuka T, Feinstone SM. Plasmid DNA-based immunization for hepatitis C virus structural proteins: immune responses in mice. *Gastroenterology* 1997; 112: 1321-30.

Outcome of surgery for colitis

N.S. Williams

Academic Department of Surgery, St Bartholomew's and the Royal London School of Medicine and Dentistry, London, United Kingdom

The patient is a female aged 30 years and has had ulcerative colitis for 12 years. The disease involves the whole colon, and her symptoms have recently been uncontrollable on oral steroids, hydrocortisone enemas, mesalazine and azathioprine. In addition, biopsies on two different occasions separated by three months confirm that she has severe dysplasia. There is little argument that this patient merits surgery; the only question is which procedure should be performed.

There are three possibilities:
1) proctocolectomy and ileostomy,
2) colectomy and ileorectal anastomosis (IRA),
3) restorative proctocolectomy (RP).

The advantages of proctocolectomy are that all the disease can be removed, but the disadvantages include possible pelvic nerve damage with bladder and sexual function being disturbed, a perineal wound which can take months to heal, and the psychological and functional disturbances attributable to a permanent ileostomy.

Colectomy and ileorectal anastomosis have the advantage of restoring gastrointestinal continuity and continence. However, disease is left behind in the rectum which can cause continuing symptoms, not only in relation to bowel function, but also because of systemic problems, such as arthropathy and skin disease. The main disadvantage of leaving behind diseased rectal mucosa, especially when dysplasia is present, is the risk of rectal cancer. In patients in whom dysplasia is not present, this risk has been shown to be 6% at 20 years and 15% at 30 years [1]. In the patient with dysplasia, there can be little argument that IRA is contra-indicated. Even if dysplasia was not present, we would argue that the risk should not be taken in this young patient with the rest of her life to lead.

The third option, and the one we would favour, would be restorative proctocolectomy (RP). To appreciate the arguments, it is necessary first to understand how this procedure developed and how it is performed today. The operation was first described by Sir Alan Parks in 1978. His concept was that ulcerative colitis was a mucosal disease. If, therefore, a colectomy was performed and the rectal mucosa was removed by mucosectomy, all the disease could be eliminated. Gastrointestinal continuity could then be restored by fashioning a pouch from the terminal ileum, thus creating a neorectum which could be drawn down through the denuded rectal muscular cuff and anastomosed transanally to the dentate line *(figure 1)*. A defunctioning ileostomy was constructed to allow the pouch and anastomosis to heal, and the ileostomy was closed 6-8 weeks later when a water soluble contrast enema showed no evidence of leakage. The original technique was tedious to perform, especially the mucosectomy, and often led to sepsis developing between the rectal muscular cuff and the pouch. Hence, the length of cuff was gradually reduced in length, eventually being no longer than 5 cm from the anal verge *(figure 2)*. However, because the anastomosis had to be performed transanally with stretching of the anal sphincter, continence was far from perfect. With the introduction of stapling instruments, a totally stapled technique was next introduced [2]. This had the advantage of creating an anastomosis without damage to the anal sphincter. In addition, it was technically easier to perform, and hence reduced the time of the operation considerably. It is now the technique that is used most frequently, usually accompanied by formation of a J pouch *(figure 3)*. Its disadvantage is that a mucosectomy is not performed, and invariably 1-2 cm of rectum is left above the dentate line which may be diseased, and in our patient may be dysplastic. Thus, the correct operation in our patient should be a restorative proctocolectomy with a mucosectomised short cuff of rectum with a transanal pouch-anal anastomosis being performed at the dentate line. Such a procedure trades off optimum function for virtual elimination of the cancer risk provided an accurate and complete mucosectomy can be performed. On the other hand, if our patient did not have dysplasia, it would be reasonable to perform a totally stapled RP with no mucosectomy. Although we would favour a restorative proctocolectomy in our patient, it is essential to counsel the patient carefully and offer as an alternative a proctocolectomy and permanent ileostomy. Despite the downside of an ileostomy, as previously mentioned, it is a one-stage operation and is not marred by frequency of defaecation and possible continence problems. In order to counsel the patient satisfactorily about the pros and cons of restorative proctocolectomy, it is important to understand the results that can be achieved with such a procedure and the complications that might ensue.

The early complications are listed in *table I*. Fortunately, the risk of death is small *(table II)*. The commonest problems are intestinal obstruction and pelvic sepsis. Obstruction varies from approximately 6-31%, but surgery is rarely required [3-8] *(table III)*. Pelvic sepsis can result from haemorrhage or anastomotic leakage and occurs in approximately 4-17% of cases and decreases with the surgeon's experience *(table IV)*. Various factors can affect anastomotic leakage and pelvic sepsis and these include age, sex, steroids, severity of rectal disease, staging of the procedure, perianal disease, type of anastomosis and whether a covering stoma has been used. Late complications include sexual and bladder dysfunction, anastomotic stricture, poor anorectal function and pouchitis *(table V)*. The autonomic nerves to the pelvis are at risk in any operation in which the rectum is excised. Provided that a close perimuscular rectal dissection is performed, these risks should be reduced. In males the risk of impotence and retrograde ejaculation is less than

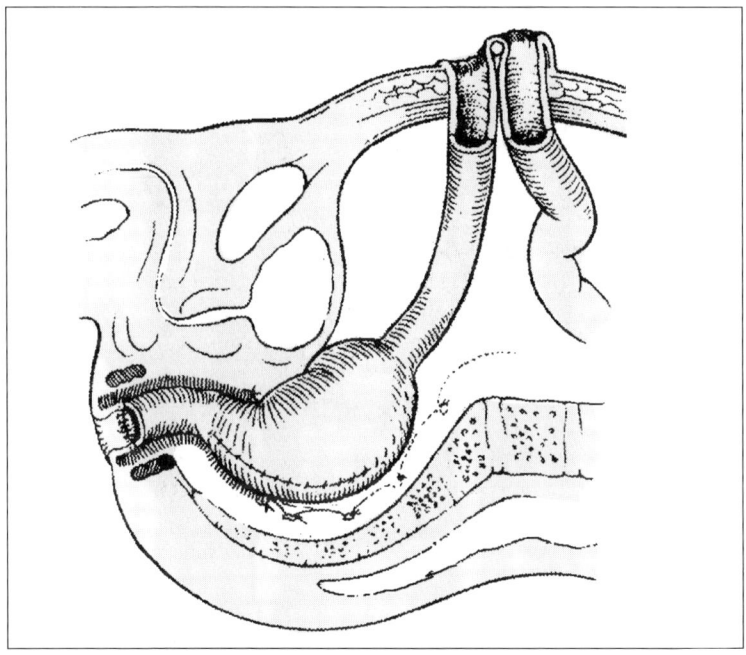

Figure 1. Restorative proctocolectomy. Original procedure described by Parks [34]. Note the long mucosectomised rectal cuff.

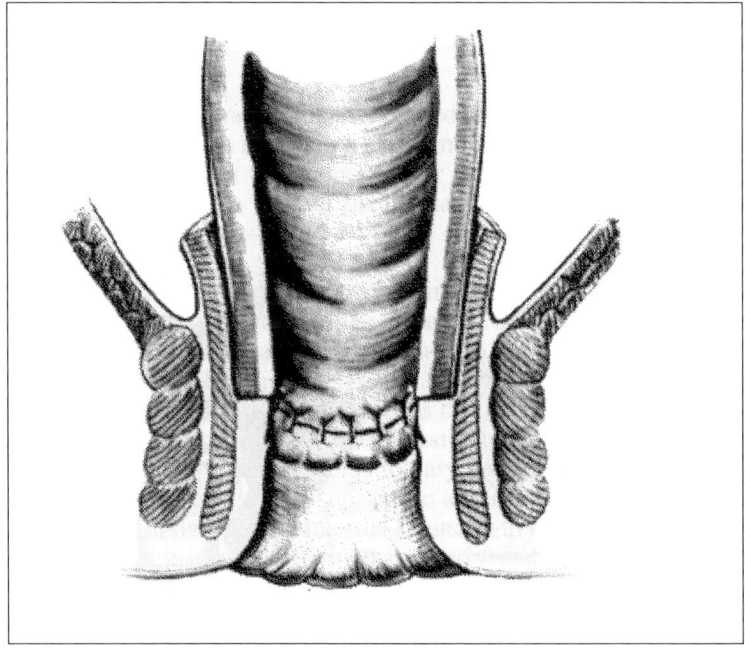

Figure 2. Restorative proctocolectomy with short mucosectomised cuff.

References

1. Baker WNW, Glass RE, Ritchie JK, Aylett SO. Cancer of the rectum following colectomy and ileorectal anastomosis for ulcerative colitis. *Br J Surg* 1978; 65: 862-8.
2. Heald RJ, Allen DR. Stapled ileoanal anastomosis; a technique to avoid mucosal proctectomy in the ileal pouch operation. *Br J Surg* 1986; 73: 571-2.
3. Schoetz DJ, Coller JA, Veidenheimer MC. Ileoanal reservoir for ulcerative colitis and familial polyposis. *Arch Surg* 1986; 121: 404-9.
4. Fonkalsrud EW. Update on clinical experience with different surgical techniques of the endorectal pull-through operation for colitis and polyposis. *Surg Gynaecol Obstet* 1987; 165: 309-16.
5. Oresland T, Fasth S, Nordgren S, Hulten L. The clinical and functional outcome after restorative proctocolectomy. A prospective study in 100 patients. *Int J Colorectal Dis* 1989; 4: 50-6.
6. Williams NS, Dozois RR, Goldberg SM, *et al*. Restorative proctocolectomy with ileal reservoir. *Int J Colorectal Dis* 1986; 1: 2-16.
7. Sagar PM, Holdsworth PJ, King RFGJ, Salter G, Johnston D. Single lumen ileum with myectomy: a possible alternative to the pelvic reservoir in restorative proctocolectomy. *Br J Surg* 1990; 77: 1030-5.
8. Keighley MRB, Grobler S, Bain I. An audit of restorative proctocolectomy. *Gut* 1993; 34: 680-4.
9. McHugh SM, Diamant NE, McLeod R, Cohen Z. S pouches *vs* J pouches. A comparison of functional outcomes. *Dis Colon Rectum* 1987; 30: 671-7.
10. Skarsgard ED, Atkinson KG, Bell GA, Pezim ME, Seal AM, Sharp FR. Function and quality of life results after ileal pouch surgery for chronic ulcerative colitis and familial polyposis. *Am J Surg* 1989; 157: 467-71.
11. Wexner SD, Jensen L, Rothenberger DA, Wong WD, Goldberg SM. Long-term functional analysis of the ileoanal reservoir. *Dis Colon Rectum* 1989; 32: 275-81.
12. Cohen Z, McLeod RS, Stern H, *et al*. The pelvic pouch and ileoanal anastomosis procedure: surgical technique and initial results. *Am J Surg* 1985; 150: 601-7.
13. Pezim ME, Nicholls RJ. Quality of life after restorative proctocolectomy with pelvic ileal reservoir. *Br J Surg* 1985; 12: 31-3.
14. Becker JM, Raymond JL. Ileal pouch-anal anastomosis: a single surgeon's experience with 100 consecutive cases. *Ann Surg* 1986; 204: 375-83.
15. Nasmyth DG, Johnston D, Godwin PGR, Dixon MR, Smith A, Williams NS. Factors influencing bowel function after ileal pouch-anal anastomosis. *Br J Surg* 1986; 73: 469-73.
16. Pemberton JH, Kelly KA, Beart RW Jr, Dozois RR, Wolff BG, Ilstrup DM. Ileal pouch-anal anastomosis for chronic ulcerative colitis – long term results. *Ann Surg* 1987; 206: 504-11.
17. Corry DG, Bond C, Jones D, Notter J, Williams NS. A nationwide survey of the functional results of restorative proctocolectomy. *Br J Surg* 1997; Suppl 84: 26.
18. Nicholls RJ, Holt SDH, Lubowski DZ. Restorative proctocolectomy with ileal reservoir. Comparison of two-stage vs three-stage procedures and analysis of factors that might affect outcome. *Dis Colon Rectum* 1989; 32: 323-6.
19. Metcalf AM, Dozois RR, Kelly KA. Sexual function in women with proctocolectomy. *Ann Surg* 1986; 204: 624-7.
20. Nelson H, Dozois RR, Kelly KA, Malkasian GD, Wolff BG, Ilstrup DM. The effect of pregnancy and delivery on the ileal pouch anal anastomosis function. *Dis Colon Rectum* 1989; 32: 384-8.
21. Snooks SJ, Setchell M, Swash M, Henry MM. Injury to the innervation of the pelvic floor sphincter musculature in childbirth. *Lancet* 1984; 546-50.
22. Mortensen NJMcC. Patient selection for restorative proctocolectomy. In: Nicholls J, Bartolo D, Mortensen N, eds. *Restorative proctocolectomy*. Blackwell Scientific Publications, 1993; 7-17.
23. Dozois RR. Ileal "J" pouch-anal anastomosis. *Br J Surg* 1985; 72 (suppl): 580-2.

24. Telander RL, Spencer M, Perrault J, Telander D, Zinsmeister AR. Long term follow-up of the ileoanal anastomosis in children and young adults. *Surgery* 1990; 108: 717-25.
25. Deutsch A, McLeod RS, Cullen J, Cohen Z. Results of the pelvic pouch procedure in patients with Crohn's disease. *Dis Colon Rectum* 1991; 34: 475-7.
26. Nicholls RJ. Restorative proctocolectomy with various types of reservoir. *World J Surg* 1987; 11: 751-62.
27. Grobler S, Affice E, Keighley MRB, Thompson H. Outcome in patients with restorative proctocolectomy and a suspected diagnosis of Crohn's disease. *Br J Surg* 1991; 78: 729.
28. Hyman NH, Fazio VW, Tuckson WB, Lavery IC. The consequences of ileal pouch-anal anastomosis for Crohn's colitis. *Dis Colon Rectum* 1991; 34: 653-7.
29. Price AB. Overlap in the spectrum of non-specific inflammatory bowel disease – "colitis indeterminate". *J Clin Pathol* 1978; 31: 567-77.
30. Lee KS, Medline A, Hockey S. Indeterminate colitis in the spectrum of inflammatory bowel disease. *Arch Pathol Lab Med* 1979; 193: 173-6.
31. Pezim ME, Pemberton JH, Beart RW, *et al*. Outcome of "indeterminate" colitis following ileal pouch-anal anastomosis. *Dis Colon Rectum* 1989; 32: 653-8.
32. Wells AD, McMillan I, Price AB, Ritchie JK, Nicholls RJ. Natural history of indeterminate colitis. *Br J Surg* 1991; 78: 179-81.
33. Morgan RA, Manning PB, Coran AG. Experience with the straight endorectal pull-through for the management of ulcerative colitis and familial polyposis in children and adults. *Ann Surg* 1987; 206: 595-9.
34. Parks AG, Nicholls RJ. Quality of life after restorative proctocolectomy with pelvic ileal reservoir. *Br J Surg* 1985; 72: 31-3.

Management of pain in chronic pancreatitis

P.U. Reber, M.W. Büchler

Department of Visceral and Transplantation Surgery, Inselspital, University of Bern, Bern, Switzerland

Summary

Chronic pancreatitis is a disease characterized by irreversible destruction of the pancreas and replacement of the parenchyma by dense fibrous tissue. The most common aetiological factor (80%) in Western countries is alcohol abuse. Pain is the outstanding clinical symptom in most patients with chronic pancreatitis. Although the mechanisms of pain in chronic pancreatitis are still elusive, there is growing evidence that neuro-immune interactions may be important. A careful clinical and diagnostic investigation, including CT scanning and endoscopic retrograde cholangio-pancreatography (ERCP), is mandatory in these patients in order to determine the need for further treatment. In the absence of major morphologic lesions of the pancreatic duct or pancreatic parenchyma, conservative treatment is advised. This includes abstinence from alcohol, analgesics, diet and enzyme replacement. In the presence of complications, such as intractable pain, which is usually caused by pancreatic head enlargement, stenosis of the common bile duct and/or the pancreatic duct, pseudocysts or inability to exclude pancreatic cancer, surgery is recommended. Among the various surgical procedures, ranging from drainage operations to partial pancreaticoduodenectomies, the duodenum-preserving resection of the head of the pancreas (DPRHP) is considered the most physiological approach and has several advantages in terms of decreased postoperative endocrine deterioration, less pain, better weight gain and less gastric emptying delay, compared with other surgical procedures. The role of interventional procedures such as stenting of pancreatic duct, bile duct or pseudocyst drainage has yet to be determined.

Chronic pancreatitis is characterized by painful progressive loss of exocrine and endocrine tissue. The most common cause of chronic pancreatitis worldwide is alcohol [1]. Idiopathic and tropical pancreatitis constitutes the remainder of cases [2]. Although pain is the most common symptom, chronic pancreatitis can be clinically silent in some patients. Similarly, many patients with unexplained abdominal pain may have chronic pancreatitis that eludes diagnosis. The true prevalence of the disease is therefore not known, although estimates range from 0.04 to 5% [3]. In some countries, the incidence of chronic pancreatitis has increased over the last 40-years [4]. The significance of these data, however, is uncertain. The trend may represent increased awareness and diagnostic ability, rather than a real change in disease epidemiology [5].

The aim of all therapeutic approaches in chronic pancreatitis is of pain relief and preservation of exocrine and endocrine pancreatic function. Despite the fact that chronic pancreatitis is a disease which should be treated conservatively, almost every second patient with chronic pancreatitis will undergo surgery during the course of the disease for intractable pain, or for complications [6]. There has been considerable debate concerning whether the pain of chronic pancreatitis can be expected to diminish with time. Amman et al. [7] followed 145 patients with alcoholic pancreatitis for a median of 10.4 years and found that 85% experienced lasting pain relief irrespective as to whether they were treated conservatively, or with surgery. This study has promoted the concept that in a substantial number of patients, chronic pancreatitis will eventually "burn itself out" with lasting pain relief and that surgery is of questionable value in the management of chronic pain. A critical analysis of this study shows that the patients coming to surgery were a selected group because they were failures of conservative management. Most of the operations performed in these patients would no longer be considered appropriate. Additionally, pain in chronic pancreatitis needs active, either conservative or operative, treatment and it seems unethical to wait until chronic pancreatitis eventually burns itself out, a process which may take years. In the meantime the psychological and socioeconomic consequences of severe chronic pancreatitis are almost invariably disastrous and the long-term mortality is high, often from the consequences of alcohol abuse, opiate dependency or suicide. The first choice in patients with chronic pancreatitis is still conservative treatment. Nevertheless, its predominant position in patients with abnormal CT or ERCP findings corresponding to morphological lesions has been challenged by newer, more physiological operative methods, namely the duodenum-preserving resection of the head of the pancreas (DPRHP). This operation has shown excellent long-term results with a low mortality and morbidity in experienced hands. Büchler et al. [8] reported that of 298 patients undergoing a DPRHP 88% were pain free or had only occasional pain not needing treatment after a median follow-up of 6 years: 63% of the patients were able to return to work. In-hospital mortality in this study was 1%. Additionally, operative treatment may also retard the progression of exo-and endocrine insufficiency [9, 10].

Pathogenesis of chronic pancreatitis

The mechanism by which alcohol induces chronic pancreatitis is still a matter of dispute. Several theories are under discussion (table I). Sarles' theory proposes that the initial step is a primary effect of alcohol on pancreatic exocrine secretion, with protein plug formation and obstruction of intrapancreatic ductules. Some data support the concept that a specific "pancreatic stone protein", known as PSP (or lithostatin), plays a central role in preventing precipitation of calcium salts. Low PSP levels could therefore favour the formation of intraductal calcification, with subsequent focal obstruction and the patchy lobular distri-

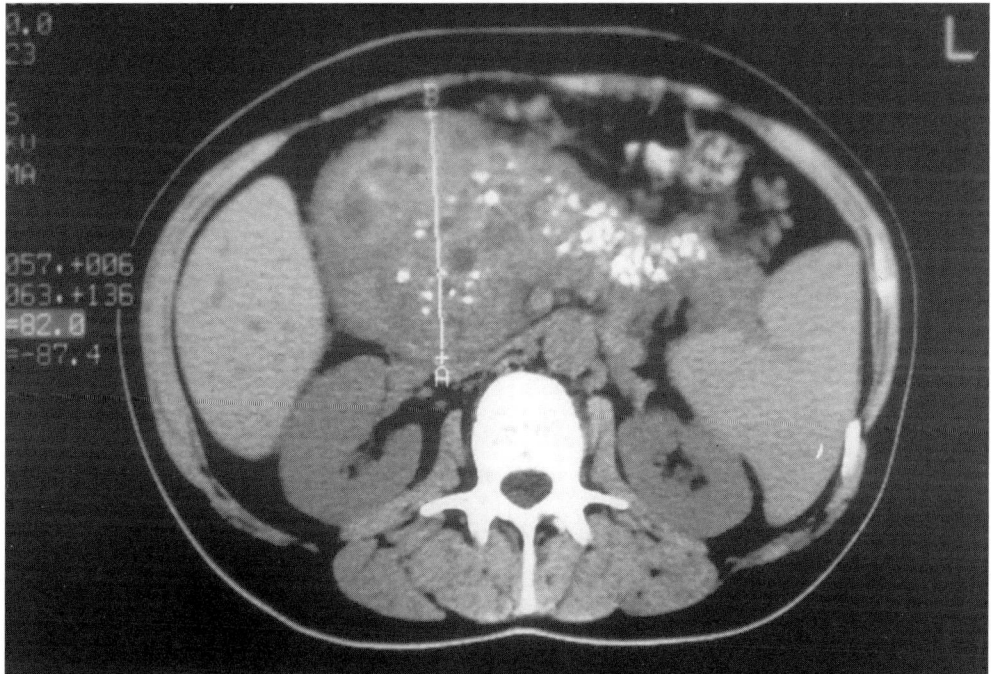

Figure 1. CT scan of a patient with severe calcific chronic pancreatitis and massive pancreatic head enlargement.

Table I. Different pathogenic concepts of chronic pancreatitis

Author	Concept
Sarles et al [11]	Intraductal protein plugs due to low levels of « pancreatic stone protein »
Bardolo et al [14]	Disordered hepatic detoxification
Braganza et al [15]	Fatty degeneration of pancreatic cells, associated with loss of zymogen content and peri acinar fibrosis
Kloeppel et al [16-18] Hunger et al [19] Friess et al [20] Kashiwagi et al [21]	Recurrent bouts of acute pancreatitis, fibrosis-necrosis sequence Cell mediated cytotoxicity Enhanced urokinase plasminogen activation Altered phospholipase A2 activation

bution of inflammation which characterizes chronic pancreatitis. According to Sarles' et al. [11] the formation of these calcium precipitates due to a decreased synthesis of PSP is the key initial lesion in the pathogenesis of chronic pancreatitis. The theory is supported by the observation that the amount of messenger RNA encoding for PSP is lower in the juice and acini of patients with chronic calcific pancreatitis than in controls, regardless of whether the disease is alcoholic, hereditary, tropical, or idiopathic in origin [12]. In contrast to Sarles' hypothesis which considers acinar cell damage to be primarily due to ductular

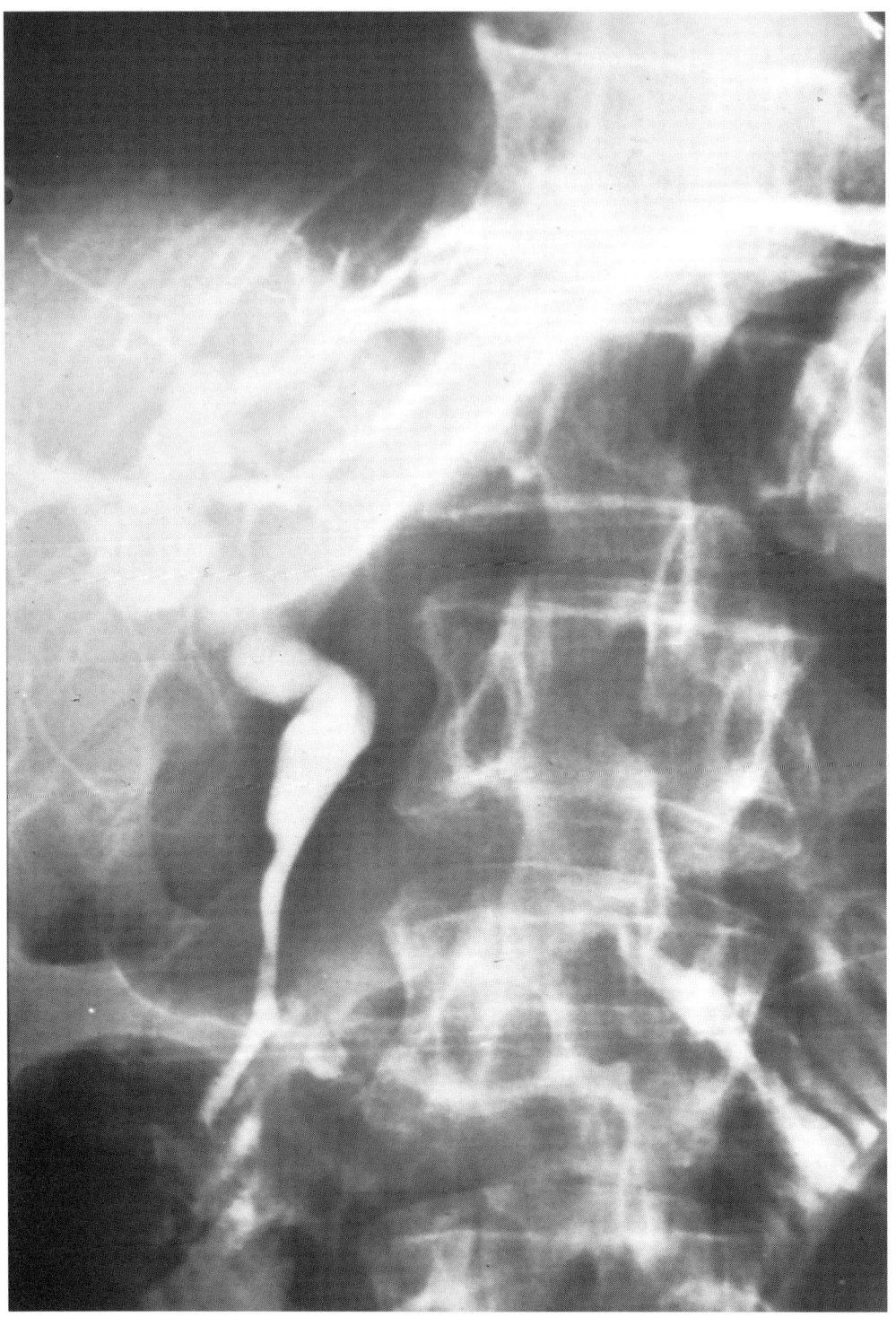
Figure 2. ERCP of the same patient showing stenosis of the distal common bile duct.

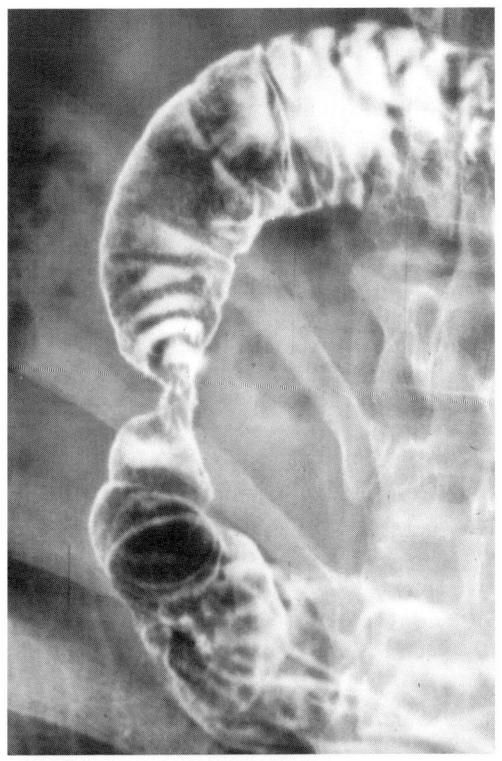

Figure 3. Hypotonic duodenography in a patient with chronic pancreatitis, demonstrating severe stenosis of the duodenum.

obstruction by protein precipitates, others have suggested that these changes are secondary to fatty degeneration of pancreatic cells, associated with loss of zymogen content and periacinar fibrosis [13, 14]. It has been postulated that overstimulation of the acinar cells could derange intracellular transport of secretory proteins with abnormal admixture of digestive enzymes and lysosomal hydrolases and/or storage of zymogens in acid compartments. Additionally, alcohol may lead to the production of toxic metabolites of lipid metabolism in pancreatic cells and trigger the development of chronic pancreatitis. Yet another hypothesis is that disordered hepatic detoxification is the prime initiator of chronic pancreatitis [15]. This concept is based on the finding that alcohol can induce hepatic mixed function oxidases. The process may be facilitated by an abundant intake of unsaturated fatty acids and could depend on individual genetic predisposition. According to this hypothesis, products of hepatic detoxification, such as oxygen free radicals and reactive toxic intermediates, are then excreted into the bile and could cause damage to the pancreas after regurgitation into the duct system. Kloeppel *et al.* [16-18] proposed a hypothesis that relates the pathogenesis of chronic pancreatitis to that of acute pancreatitis. In their opinion, the basic pathogenic event in the evolution of chronic pancreatitis is a necrosis-fibrosis sequence due to recurrent bouts of acute pancreatitis. This implies that acute pancreatitis, probably in its severe relapsing form, may be the cause of chronic pancreatitis. Recent work from our laboratory adds additional weight to this theory. Hunger *et al.* [19] observed increased frequency of perforin mRNA-expressing cells in chronic pancreatitis indicating a preferential activation of these effector cells of cell-mediated cytotoxicity. The close association between activated cytotoxic cells with remaining intact pancreatic parenchyma indicate that these cells are directly involved in the destruction of parenchymal cells. It also provides circumstantial evidence for involvement of autoreactive cytotoxic T cells and NK cells in the pathogenesis of this disease. Friess et al. [20] showed that urokinase plasminogen activator, responsible for the regulation of plasmin generation from plasminogen, and its receptor contribute to the lytic damage observed in chronic pancreatitis by plasmin generation and that increased amounts of plasmin activate latent TGF-β, thereby leading to the accumulation of fibrotic tissue. Similarly, Kashiwagi et al. [21] demonstrated an upregulation of the phospholipase A2 (PLA2) isoforms type II and type IV in the presence of decreased phospholipase type I. PLA2 type I is usually elevated in patients with acute pancreatitis, whereas PLA2 type II has mitogenic effects on fibroblasts and PLA2 type IV is transcriptionally upregulated in fibroblasts. These findings are also consistent with the process of ongoing inflammatory damage and remodeling of pancreatic parenchyma.

Regardless of the aetiology of chronic pancreatitis, one common histological finding apart from the marked fibrosis is that chronic inflammatory cells cluster around nerves in and around the pancreas, inducing damage to the perineurium and eventually affecting nerve fibres.

Mechanisms of pain in chronic pancreatitis

The presence of pain in chronic pancreatitis is well known. However, the pathogenesis has not been fully worked out, although several theories have been proposed *(table II)*. It must be accepted that the perception of pain depends on impulses carried by nerves to appropriate locations in the central nervous system.

Table II. Mechanisms of pain in chronic pancreatitis

- Pancreatic duct obstruction
- Pseudocysts
- Activation of stretch receptors (pancreatic swelling)
- Reduction of pancreatic blood flow with consequent ischemia
- Bile duct obstruction, duodenal obstruction
- Neuro-immune interaction

It is well known that when stretch receptors in the gastrointestinal tract are stimulated, pain may be experienced. The pain that some patients experience during ERCP [22] is an indication that stretch receptors may be involved in pain production in the pancreas. Thus it is reasonable to question whether pain is produced by higher pressures of pancreatic juice within the ductal system in chronic pancreatitis. There is good evidence that pressures are elevated in chronic pancreatitis. Bradley et al. [23] reported the intrapancreatic ductal pressure was significantly elevated in patients with chronic pancreatitis. The clinical impression of correlation of pain severity with higher pressure has been reported [23]. In experimental studies [24] it has been shown that, under conditions of chronic pancreatitis or artificial limitation of tissue expansion, interstitial pressure increases secondary to elevated ductal pressures. Manes et al. [25] found that the interstitial pressure in the pancreas of patients with chronic pancreatitis was significantly higher than in controls, but without correlation between parenchymal pressure and pain. Patel et al. [26] suggested that the increased interstitial pressure is responsible for decreased pancreatic blood flow, thus causing ischaemic pain. Ductal hypertension could also be caused by increased secretion and/or decreased outflow. It has been suggested that pancreatic ductal hypertension is secondary to pancreatic outflow obstruction. Malfertheiner et al. [27] measured pain after reducing pancreatic secretion in patients with chronic pancreatitis. They found no difference in pain scores, or in the consumption of analgesics, although secretion was strongly inhibited. Other causes of pain in patients with chronic pancreatitis include acute attacks of inflammation of the pancreas, which presumably involves similar mechanisms as those associated with acute pancreatitis [28]. Stenosis of the distal common bile duct has been noted to be associated with severe abdominal pain. While this pain might be caused by distension of the common bile duct, pain might also be caused by an associated duodenal stenosis [29]. It is likely that multiple factors are involved in the generation of pain. Although it is tempting to ascribe one mechanism for initiating and sustaining pancreatic pain, it should be recognized that there may be different ways of stimulating an intact nervous complex in a manner perceived as pain. Furthermore, the nervous complex of the pancreas may change as the disease develops.

There is accumulating evidence from the initial work of Bockman et al. [30] that in chronic pancreatitis there are major abnormalities in and around the nerves. These workers have shown increased numbers and diameters of pancreatic nerve fibres in chronic pancreatitis, compared with the normal pancreas. Additional immunohistochemical studies have shown increased amounts of neurotransmitters, such as substance P, in afferent pancreatic nerves of patients with chronic pancreatitis [31]. In further studies Weihe et al. [32] and Büchler et al. [33] have shown that the pattern of intrinsic and possibly extrinsic inervation of the pancreas changes in chronic pancreatitis, leading to a differential expression of neuropeptides. Di Sebastiano et al. [34] demonstrated for the first time a direct correlation between the degree of perineural inflammation and pain. They found increased cytoplasmic expression and intensified GAP-43 (growth-associated protein 43) immunoreactivity in interlobular and intralobular pancreatic nerves, indicating changes in the intrinsic nervous system during chronic pancreatitis. This situation can be compared with a transection of peripheral nerve, which is the classic model for induction of GAP-43 expression in peripheral neurons. Interestingly, the increase of GAP-43 was found in pancreatic nerve fibres (axons of postganglionic parasympathetic neurons and fibres of extrinsic origin) and in intrinsic neurons. All subpopulations of neurons, including the afferent nociceptive fibres, are affected by the inflammation. Additionally, GAP-43 expression is dependant on the duration of the disease. Long term inflammation correlated with highest degrees of GAP-43 expression.

Clinical picture and complications in chronic pancreatitis

Although pain is the outstanding symptom in patients with chronic pancreatitis, the occurrence of painful chronic pancreatitis is variable and related to the aetiology of the disease [35]. Eighty percent of patients who have idiopathic pancreatitis with onset before the age of 36 years have moderate, or severe pain. By contrast, 46% of patients with late onset idiopathic pancreatitis have no pain. The distribution of pain in patients with alcoholic pancreatitis falls between these two types of idiopathic pancreatitis; at the time of diagnosis 23% have no pain.

There are two patterns of pain in chronic pancreatitis. Most patients have relapsing attacks that occur at very variable intervals from weekly to once every several years. Constant abdominal pain is not frequent, but difficult to manage conservatively. A complication has to be ruled out if a patient who had mild and relapsing pain suddenly develops constant daily pain. The most common causes of constant abdominal pain in these patients include a pseudocyst with an incidence between 40-60% [36], an inflammatory mass (usually in the head of the pancreas) in 50% [37], obstruction of the intrapancreatic portion of the common bile duct by the cicatricial reaction secondary to chronic pancreatitis in 9% [6], pancreatic duct obstruction in more than 50% [38], portal vein encasement in 10% [39] and duodenal stenosis in 6% of the patients [40] *(table III)*.

Table III. Complications in chronic pancreatitis

Complications	Prevalence [Ref.]
Pain	54-80% [35]
Pseudocysts	40-60% [36]
Inflammatory head enlargement	49% [37]
Pancreatic duct obstruction	>50% [38]
Suspicion of cancer	15% [43]
Hemorrhage	2-10% [42]
Common bile duct obstruction	9% [6]
Duodenal obstruction	6% [40]
Portal vein encasement	5-10% [39]
Pancreatic ascites	1% [42]
Splenic vein thrombosis	-

External pancreatic fistula as a complication of chronic pancreatitis is unusual and occurs most commonly following surgical, or percutaneous external drainage of a pseudocyst. Pancreatic ascites is a consequence of leakage of pancreatic juice from a pseudocyst, or the pancreatic duct. This occurs in 1% of patients with chronic pancreatitis and is typically found in alcoholic cirrhotics [41].

Chronic pancreatitis is the most common cause of splenic vein thrombosis [42]. This creates a segmental form of portal hypertension, which may result in gastric varices that can bleed. However, haemorrhage in chronic pancreatitis usually originates in pseudoaneurysms that involve the splenic, gastroduodenal, or pancreaticoduodenal arteries. These are commonly found in association with pseudocysts and can rupture into the cyst or into the pancreatic duct. The difficulty of excluding a carcinoma in a patient supposedly suffering from chronic pancreatitis continues to confront surgeons and physicians despite the advances in radiological methods. In about 15% of patients with chronic pancreatitis, the presence of a cancer cannot be ruled out [43].

Treatment of pain in chronic pancreatitis

Pain relief in patients with chronic pancreatitis without morphological lesions, or complications of the disease, may be achieved by conservative measures in the majority of patients. The logical use of these measures are summarized in *figure 4*.

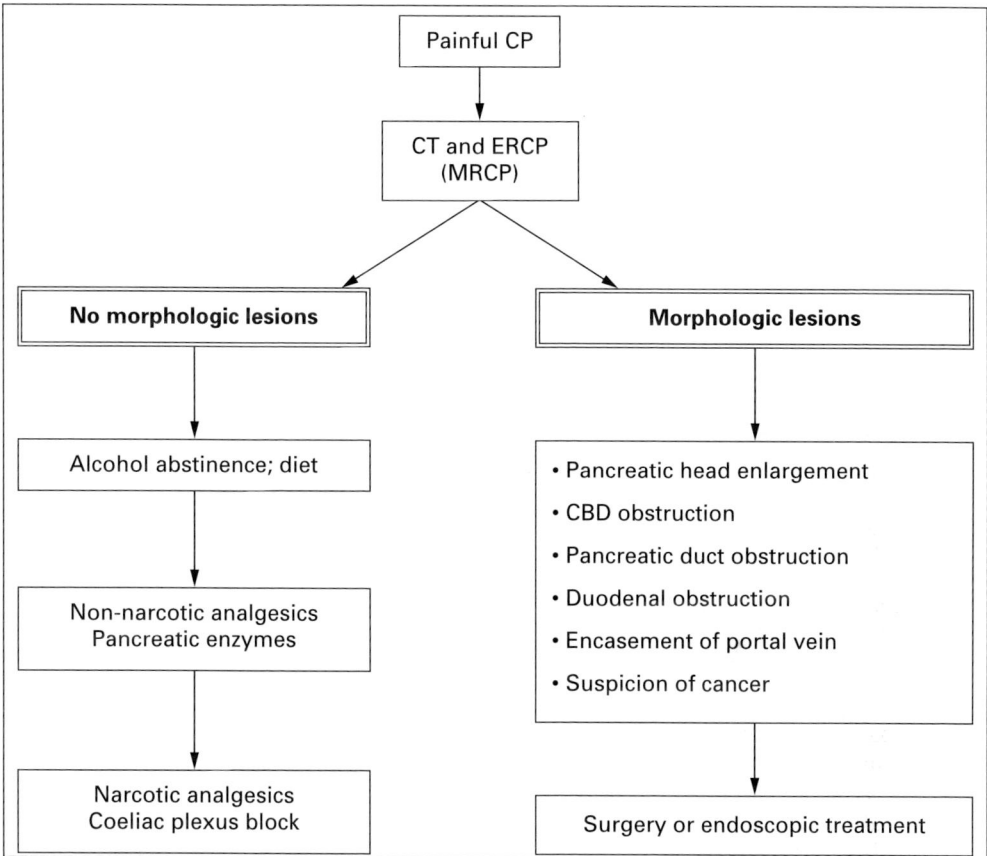

Figure 4. Algorithm for assessment and treatment of pain in chronic pancreatitis.

The first step in the management of patients with chronic pancreatitis is avoidance of alcohol *(table IV)*. Total abstinence from alcohol achieves pain relief in up to 50% of patients, mainly in those with mild or moderate disease [44]. This measure avoids the secretagogue effect of alcohol and slows down pancreatic damage [45]. No other dietetic measure has been shown to influence the course of pain in chronic pancreatitis. However, some authors recommend a restricted fat intake in order to limit the postprandial pancreatic stimulation.

Analgesic treatment should begin with non-narcotic agents (paracetamol, NSAIDs), but opioid analgesics (buprenorphin) are often required. Type and doses of analgesic drugs

Table IV. Treatment options in chronic pancreatitis

Conservative treatment of pain	• Abstinence from alcohol • Enzyme administration: only useful in early stage CP [47, 48] • Diet: low fat/high protein • Analgesics: 1) non-narcotic agents (paracetamol, NSAID's) 2) opioid analgesics • Inhibition of pancreatic secretion: only useful in selected patients [27] • Endoscopic treatment: endoscopic sphincterotomy, stenting, stone removal • Coeliac plexus block

Surgical treatment	• Drainage procedures: (pancreaticojejunostomies, Partington-Rochelle)
	• Resections: 1) duodenum-preserving resection of the head of the pancreas [58]
	             2) limited resection of the head of the pancreas
	             3) pancreatoduodenectomy with or without preservation of the pylorus [57]
	             4) total pancreatectomy

vary and treatment should be individually prescribed, using the lowest dose needed to control pain.

Based on the hypothesis that pain in chronic pancreatitis is secondary to ductal hypertension, inhibition of pancreatic secretion leading to a decrease of intraductal pressure should lead to pain relief. A protease-mediated negative feedback of exocrine pancreatic secretion has been demonstrated in humans [46]. Based on this evidence, exogenous pancreatic enzymes can be used in patients with chronic pancreatitis in order to inhibit pancreatic secretion and to decrease intraductal pressure. However, the role of enzyme treatment for pain in patients with chronic pancreatitis is still controversial and depends on dose, as well as on the severity of the disease [47, 48]. Although somatostatin, or its analogue octreotide, causes potent inhibition of pancreatic secretion, pain relief is usually not achieved by octreotide administration [27].

Several endoscopic techniques have been developed to alleviate the obstruction of pancreatic secretion: endoscopic sphincterotomy, stenting and endoscopic removal of pancreatic stones combined with extracorporal shock-wave lithotripsy. Several authors have reported pain relief after endoscopic treatment in patients with chronic pancreatitis [49, 50]. Before endoscopic removal pancreatic duct stones often need extracorporal shock-wave lithotripsy. This procedure may be useful in patients with chronic pancreatitis in whom pain is caused by stone-related obstruction [51, 52]. However, endoscopic threatment of chronic pancreatitis has several drawbacks. Firstly, there is important morbidity and mortality. In one series [53], 7 of 32 (22%) patients had complications (for example: abscess, acute pancreatitis, surgery required) and one patient died. An even more ominous development is the conversion of normal ducts to the appearance seen in chronic pancreatitis in up to 75% of the patients [54]. It seems that stenting the pancreatic duct to treat chronic pancreatitis, may induce it. Further clinical research is required to determine which patients will benefit the most from either surgical or endoscopic treatment and to what extent the two forms of management can coexist.

Coeliac plexus block by percutaneous injection of alcohol can be used in selected patients with painful chronic pancreatitis and without morphologic lesions. Unfortunately the duration of pain relief after the block is short lasting in most patients and reinjection is less effective and more risky [55].

If conservative treatment fails, or in the presence of complications, patients should undergo operative treatment. Surgery of chronic pancreatitis has recently evolved to a new stage of development. Drainage procedures of the main pancreatic duct (for example: Partington-Rochelle) or pseudocysts is still an important approach, but the best results can only be obtained in properly selected patients [56]. During the past 50 years pancreatic resection for pain has been based on the classical procedures of the Whipple's type resection, left sided pancreatic resection and total pancreatoduodenectomy. A radical breakthrough has recently occurred in the development of surgical techniques, such as the pylorus-preserving pancreaticoduodenectomy [57], the duodenum-preserving resection of the head of the pancreas (DPRHP) [58] and the operation which combines a longitudinal pancreaticojejunostomy with limited resection of tissue in the head of the pancreas [59]. These procedures focus on removing the principal lesion causing the symptoms, whilst aiming to preserve the maximum of residual pancreatic, and adjacent organ function [60-62]. DPRHP has been shown in several studies to have advantages compared to Whipple resection (with or without preservation of the pylorus), in terms of postoperative quality of life, glucose metabolism, weight gain and control of gastric emptying. This operation appears therefore to be very useful in the treatment of pain and complications of chronic pancreatitis accompanied by enlargement of the head of the pancreas.

References

1. Durbec JP, Sarles H. Multicenter survey of the etiology of pancreatic diseases. Relationship between the relative risk of developing chronic pancreatitis and alcohol, protein and lipid consumption. *Digestion* 1978; 18: 337-50.
2. Müller MK, Singer MV. Aetiology and pathogenesis of chronic pancreatitis. In: Trede M, Carter DC, eds. *Surgery of the pancreas*. Edinburgh: Churchill Livingstone, 1993: 263-71.
3. Worning H. Incidence and prevalence of chronic pancreatitis. In: Beger HG, Büchler MW, Ditschuneit H, *et al.*, eds. *Chronic pancreatitis*. Berlin: Springer, 1990: 8-13.
4. Johnson CD, Hosking S. National statistics for diet, alcohol consumption and chronic pancreatitis in England and Wales 1960-1988. *Gut* 1991; 32: 1401-5.
5. Owyang C, Levitt M. Chronic pancreatitis. In: Yamada T, Alpers DH, Owyang C, *et al.*, eds. *Textbook of gastroenterology*. Vol. 2. New York: JB Lippincott, 1991: 1874-93.
6. Trede M, Carter DC. Preoperative assessment and indications for operation in chronic pancreatitis. In: Trede M, Carter DC, eds. *Surgery of the pancreas*. Edinburgh: Churchill Livingstone, 1993: 283-97.
7. Amman RW, Akovbiantz A, Largiader F, *et al.* Course and outcome of chronic pancreatitis. Longitudinal study of a mixed medical-surgical series of 245 patients. *Gastroenterolgy* 1984; 86: 820-8.
8. Büchler MW, Friess H, Beger HA, *et al.* Duodenum-preserving pancreatic head resection: long term results. *J Gastroint Surg* 1997; 1: 13-9.
9. Nealon WH, Thompson JC. Progessive loss of pancreatic function in chronic pancreatitis is delayed by a main pancreatic duct decompression: a longitudinal prospective analysis of the modified puestow procedure. *Ann Surg* 1993; 217: 458-66.
10. Nealon WH, Townsend CM, Thompson JC. Operative drainage of the pancreatic duct delays functional impairment in patients with chronic pancreatitis: a prospective analysis. *Ann Surg* 1988; 208: 321-9.

11. Sarles H, Bernhard JP, Gullo L. Pathogenesis of chronic pancreatitis. *Gut* 1990; 31: 629-32.
12. Giorgi D, Bernhard JP, Sarles H, *et al.* Secretory pancreatic stone protein messenger RNA. Nucleotide sequence and expression in chronic calcifying pancreatitis. *J Clin Invest* 1989; 84: 100-6.
13. Noronha M, Bordalo, Dreiling DA. Alcohol and the pancreas. *Am J Gastroenterol* 1981; 76: 120-4.
14. Bordalo O, Baptista A, Dreiling DA, *et al.* Early pathomorphological pancreatic changes in chronic alcoholism. In: Gyr KE, Singer MV, Sarles H, eds. *Pancreatitis: concepts and classification.* Excerpta Medica, International Congress Series No 642. Amsterdam: Elsevier, 1954.
15. Braganza JM. Pancreatic disease: a casualty of hepatic detoxification? *Lancet* 1983; 2: 1000-3.
16. Kloeppel G, Maillet B. The morphologic basis for the evolution of acute pancreatitis into chronic pancreatitis. In: Beger HG, Büchler MW, Malfertheiner P, eds. *Standards in pancreatic surgery.* Berlin: Springer, 1993: 290-6.
17. Kloeppel G. Pathology of chronic pancreatitis and pancreatic pain. *Acta Chir Scand* 1990; 156: 261-5.
18. Kloeppel G, Maillet B. Pseudocysts in chronic pancreatitis: a morphological analysis of 57 resection specimens and 9 autopsy pancreata. *Pancreas* 1991; 6: 266-74.
19. Hunger RE, Mueller CH, Büchler MW. Cytotoxic cells are activated in cellular infiltrates of alcoholic chronic pancreatitis. *Gastroenterology* 1997; 112: 1656-63.
20. Friess H, Cantero D, Büchler MW. Enhanced urokinase plasminogen activation in chronic pancreatitis suggests a role in its pathogenesis. *Gastroenterology* 1997, in press.
21. Kashiwagi M, Friess H, Büchler MW. Phospholipase A2 isoforms are altered in chronic pancreatitis. *Ann Surg* 1997, in press.
22. Sand J, Nordback I. Prospective randomized trial of the effect of nifedipine on pancreatic irritation after endoscopic retrograde cholangiopancreatography. *Digestion* 1993; 54: 105-11.
23. Bradley EL III. Pancreatic duct pressure in chronic pancreatitis. *Am J Surg* 1982; 144: 313-6.
24. Karanjia N, Widdison AL, Reber HA, *et al.* Pancreatic ductal and interstitial pressures in cats with chronic pancreatitis. *Dig Dis Sci* 1992; 37: 268-73.
25. Manes G, Büchler MW, Malfertheiner P, *et al.* Is increased pancreatic pressure related to pain in chronic pancreatitis? *Int J Pancreatol* 1994; 15: 113-7.
26. Patel AG, Reber PU, Reber HA, *et al.* Pancreatic interstitial pH in human and feline chronic pancreatitis. *Gastroenterology* 1995; 109: 1639-45.
27. Malfertheiner P, Mayer D, Büchler MW. Treatment of pain in chronic pancreatitis by inhibition of pancreatic secretion with octreotide. *Gut* 1995; 36: 450-4.
28. Banks PA. Pain in chronic pancreatitis: pathomechanism and clinical presentation. In: Beger HG, Büchler MW, Ditschuneit H, *et al.*, eds. *Chronic pancreatitis.* Berlin: Springer, 1990: 214-7.
29. Steer ML, Waxman I, Freedman S. Chronic pancreatitis. *N Engl J Med* 1995; 332: 1482-90.
30. Bockman DE, Büchler MW, Beger HG, *et al.* Analysis of nerves in chronic pancreaitis. *Gastroenterology* 1988; 94: 1459-69.
31. Büchler MW, Weihe E. Distribution of neurotransmitters in afferent human pancreatic nerves. *Digestion* 1988; 38: 8.
32. Weihe E, Büchler MW, Müller S, *et al.* Peptidergic innervation in chronic pancreatitis. In: Beger HG, Büchler MW, Ditschuneit H, *et al.*, eds. *Chronic pancreatitis.* Berlin: Springer, 1990: 88-105.
33. Büchler MW, Weihe E, Friess H, *et al.* Changes in peptidergic innervation in chronic pancreatitis. *Pancreas* 1992; 7: 183-92.
34. Di Sebastiano P, Fink T, Büchler MW. Immune cell infiltration and growth-associated protein 43 expression correlate with pain in chronic pancreatitis. *Gastroenterology* 1997; 112: 1648-55.
35. Layer P, Yamamoto H, Di Magno EP, *et al.* The different courses of early-and late-onset idiopathic and alcoholic chronic pancreatitis. *Gastroenterology* 1994; 107: 1481-7.
36. Sanfey H, Aguilar M, Jones RS. Pseudocysts of the pancreas: a review of 97 cases. *Ann Surg* 1994; 69: 661-8.

37. Schoenberg MH, Büchler MW, Beger HG, et al. Inflammatory mass in the pancreatic head associated with chronic pancreatitis. In: Beger HG, Büchler MW, Ditschuneit H, et al., eds. *Chronic pancreatitis*. Berlin: Springer, 1990: 358-63.
38. Mayedo A, Grimm H, Soehendra N. Endoscopic interventional techniques in chronic pancreatitis. In: Trede M, Carter DC, eds. *Surgery of the pancreas*. Edinburgh: Churchill Livingstone, 1993: 299-308.
39. Beger HG, Büchler MW. Duodenum-preserving resection of the head of the pancreas in chronic pancreatitis with inflammatory mass in the head. *World J Surg* 1990; 14: 83-7.
40. Bradley EL III, Clements JL Jr. Idiopathic duodenal obstruction. An unappreciated complication of pancreatitis. *Ann Surg* 1981; 193: 638-43.
41. Neoptolemos JP, Winslet MC. Pancreatic ascites. In: Beger HG, Büchler MW, Ditschuneit H, et al., eds. *Chronic pancreatitis*. Berlin, Springer, 1990: 269-79.
42. Reber HA. Complications in chronic pancreatitis. In: Beger HG, Büchler MW, Ditschuneit H, et al., eds. *Chronic pancreatitis*. Berlin: Springer, 1990: 253-5.
43. Carter DC. Cancer of the head of the pancreas or chronic pancreatitis. A diagnostic dilemma. *Surgery* 1992; 111: 602-3.
44. Strum WB. Abstinence in alcoholic chronic pancreatitis: effect on pain and outcome. *J Clin Gastroenterol* 1995; 20: 4-5.
45. Gullo L, Barbara L, Labo G. Effect of cessation of alcohol abuse on the course of pancreatic dysfunction in alcoholic pancreatitis. *Gastroenterology* 1988; 95: 1063-8.
46. Adler G, Müllenhoff A, Koop I, et al. Stimulation of pancreatic secretion in man by a protease inhibitor. *Eur J Clin Invest* 1086; 18: 98-104.
47. Mössner J, Secknus R, Meyer J, et al. Treatment of pain with pancreatic extracts in chronic pancreatitis: results of a prospective placebo-controlled multicenter trial. *Digestion* 1992; 53: 54-66.
48. Malesci A, Gaja E, Fioretta A, et al. No effect of long-term treatment with pancreatic extract on recurrent abdominal pain in patients with chronic pancreatitis. *Scand J Gastroenterol* 1995; 30: 392-8.
49. Kozarek RA, Patterson DJ, Ball TJ, et al. Endoscopic placement of pancreatic stents and drains in the management of pancreatitis. *Ann Surg* 1989; 209: 261-6.
50. Cremer M, Devière J, Delhaye M, et al. Stenting in severe chronic pancreatitis: results of a medium-term follow-up in 76 patients. *Endoscopy* 1991; 23: 171-6.
51. Delhaye M, Vandermeeren A, Cremer M, et al. Extracorporal shock-wave lithotrypsy of pancreatic calculi. *Gastroenterology* 1992; 102: 610-20.
52. Sauerbruch T, Holl J, Sackmann M, et al. Extracorporal lithotripsy of pancreatic stones in patients with chronic pancreatitis and pain. A prospective follow-up study. *Gut* 1992; 33: 969-72.
53. Huibregtse K, Schneider B, Tytgat GN, et al. Endoscopic pancreatic drainage in chronic pancreatitis. *Gastroint Endosc* 1988; 34: 9-15.
54. Kozarek RE. Pancreatic stents can induce ductal changes consistent with chronic pancreatitis. *Gastroint Endosc* 1989; 35: A170.
55. Leung JWC, Bowen-Wright M, Avelin W, et al. Coeliac plexus block for pain in pancreatic cancer and chronic pancreatitis. *Br J Surg* 1983; 70: 730-2.
56. Warshaw AL. Conservation of pancreatic tissue by combined gastric, biliary and pancreatic duct drainage for pain from chronic pancreatitis. *Am J Surg* 1985; 149: 163-9.
57. Traverso LW, Longmire WP. Preservation pylorus in the pancreaticoduodenectomy. *Surg Gynecol Obstet* 1978; 146: 956-62.
58. Beger HG, Witte C, Büchler MW. Erfahrung mit einer das Duodenum erhaltenden Pankreaskopfresektion bei chronischer Pankreatitis. *Chirurg* 1980; 51: 303-9.
59. Frey CF, Amikura K. Description and rationale of a new operation for chronic pancreatitis. *Pancreas* 1987; 2: 701-7.

60. Beger HG, Büchler MW, Bittner RR, *et al.* Duodenum-preserving resection of the head of the pancreas in severe chronic pancreatitis. *Ann Surg* 1989; 209: 273-8.
61. Müller MW, Friess H, Büchler MW. Gastric emptying following pylorus-preserving Whipple and duodenum-preserving pancreatic head resection in patients with chronic pancreatitis. *Am J Surg* 1997; 173: 257-63.
62. Büchler MW, Friess H, Müller MW, *et al.* Randomized trial of duodenum-preserving pancreatic head resection versus pylorus-preserving Whipple in chronic pancreatitis. *Am J Surg* 1995; 169: 65-70.

Management of "anismus" in adults

M.A. Kamm

Physiology Unit, St Mark's Hospital, Harrow, United Kingdom

Summary

In the mid 1980's it became apparent that many patients with the symptomatic complaint of constipation, in whom there was no apparent structural or organic abnormality, inappropriately contracted their pelvic floor during attempted defaecation. This phenomenon of "anismus", also known as "obstructed defaecation, inappropriate pelvic floor contraction, puborectalis paradoxical contraction, and recto-anal dyssynergia" was seen much more commonly in patients than in healthy control subjects. It has subsequently become apparent that the symptom of impaired evacuation almost certainly encompasses a range of causes. The term "anismus" and other similar terms imply just one particular mechanism, and for this reason I believe it is more helpful to speak of "impaired evacuation", leaving the question of pathogenic mechanism open.

In the mid 1980's it became apparent that many patients with the symptomatic complaint of constipation, in whom there was no apparent structural or organic abnormality, inappropriately contracted their pelvic floor during attempted defaecation [1]. This phenomenon of "anismus", also known as "obstructed defaecation, inappropriate pelvic floor contraction, puborectalis paradoxical contraction, and recto-anal dyssynergia" was seen much more commonly in patients than in healthy control subjects.

It has subsequently become apparent that the symptom of impaired evacuation almost certainly encompasses a range of causes. The term "anismus" and other similar terms imply just one particular mechanism, and for this reason I believe it is more helpful to speak of "impaired evacuation", leaving the question of pathogenic mechanism open.

Who suffers from impaired rectal evacuation and what causes it?

Impaired rectal evacuation occurs most commonly in women, although it can also occur in men. In most there is no obvious provoking factor, while in others there may be a precipitating event.

In some patients there may be slow colonic transit and straining occurs in a vain attempt to empty the bowel. Impaired evacuation can also coexist with anatomical abnormalities such as a large (greater than 2 cm on a lateral radiograph) rectocoele [2].

Alternatively, impaired evacuation may result from inappropriately learned defaecatory behaviour from earlier in life. Many of these patients have experienced sexual abuse early in life [3]; lack of awareness of pelvic coordination may relate to a subconscious desire by the patients to dissociate themselves from their own pelvis and genitalia.

Constipation sometimes follows pelvic surgery such as a hysterectomy. This has previously been attributed to pelvic nerve damage, but may relate to temporary interference with pelvic structures. Alternatively temporary constipation after pelvic surgery may become entrenched in a new abnormal pattern of behaviour. There may even be grief associated with hysterectomy which leads to subconscious abnormal behaviour. The successful treatment of patients with intractable constipation after hysterectomy using biofeedback techniques suggests that in some patients this is a behavioural and not a structural or neurological problem.

Testing for inappropriate pelvic floor contraction

There are several ways that such inappropriate pelvic floor contraction can be tested for:

– **Intra-anal pressure sensor**. On straining to defaecate the intra-anal pressure normally falls below that of the rectum.

– **Electromyography**. This can be a surface EMG, using skin electrodes or a plug electrode, or needle electromyography. The activity of the external sphincter and puborectalis normally inhibits during defaecation straining.

– **Evacuation proctography**. An indentation of the puborectalis muscle on the posterior wall of the rectum during attempted evacuation, together with diminished opening of the anal canal and slow, incomplete rectal emptying has been attributed to impaired anal sphincter relaxation.

– **Models of defaecation**. The ability to expel a water filled balloon from the rectum has been used to test evacuatory function.

Intrarectal pressure and external sphincter electromyography can be recorded simultaneously during evacuation proctography [4], but this has provided less additional useful information than might have been expected.

The symptom of impaired rectal evacuation has been attributed to inappropriate pelvic floor contraction. However this approach has been too simplistic, for several reasons:

(1) **The tests differ in their demonstration of this phenomenon**, with different measurement techniques of pelvic floor contraction often give conflicting results.

Miller et al. [5] studied 24 patients with constipation, 13 with measured slow transit and 11 with normal transit. Videoproctography and external sphincter electromyography were performed simultaneously – electromyographic paradoxical contraction did not consistently correlate with the ability to evacuate the rectum on proctography, or with symptoms of "obstructed defaecation".

Similar observations were reported by Wald et al. [6] who studied 36 patients with chronic constipation by evacuation proctography and anorectal manometry. Twenty patients also had a colonic transit study, 10 having normal and 10 having delayed transit. Poor rectal emptying on proctography did not correlate with a paradoxical rise in anal pressure on straining: when manometry was abnormal only one third of patients had an abnormal proctogram; conversely when manometry was normal the proctogram was also normal in 88 percent of patients.

(2) **The phenomenon is not specific to patients with a defaecation disorder**, and may involve non-defaecatory muscles.

Many patients with a variety of defaecation disorders, such as the solitary ulcer syndrome, idiopathic perineal pain [7] and even faecal incontinence [8] exhibit the same phenomenon, and it may also be observed in normal subjects. When other striated muscles, such as the external oblique and gluteus maximus, are monitored during straining, they may also contract inappropriately [9].

(3) **Patients with slow colonic transit ("idiopathic slow transit constipation") can also suffer from abnormal pelvic floor contraction** – the two conditions overlap.

(4) **Laboratory testing may not be a good reflection of real life**.

Measurements of pelvic floor activity and incoordination in the laboratory have been criticised on the basis that the patient is straining in an unnatural way, without emptying the bowel, and in a left lateral position while being observed. This may be true, although non constipated subjects observed under the same circumstances usually do relax their pelvic floor normally. Ambulatory studies of the anorectum, using solid state strain gauge transducers and fine wire electromyography of the external anal sphincter, have been undertaken in patients with constipation and pelvic floor contraction diagnosed in the laboratory. These studies have shown that when attempting to defaecate on the toilet at home many of these patients do apparently relax their pelvic floor.

Psychological aspects to impaired defaecation

Patients with impaired defaecation often have impaired psychological well being, and this may contribute to, or even be the cause of, constipation and evacuatory disturbance in some patients. In a recent study, 47 women with idiopathic constipation were compared with 28 healthy women, and 26 women with Crohn's disease, who were age-matched [10]. Patients with constipation had increased anxiety, depression, somatization and social dysfunction, and a less satisfactory sexual life, when compared to both control groups. Patients with constipation also have a higher than expected prevalence of sexual or physical abuse. These factors need to be considered as part of these patients' treatment.

Treatment

Biofeedback and habit training for idiopathic constipation

Biofeedback conditioning for constipation was originally employed in the belief that abnormal pelvic floor contraction is a learned phenomenon which causes constipation. Bleijenberg and Kuijpers [11] used an intensive in-patient regime to treat ten patients with both delayed colonic transit and abnormal pelvic floor activity. Seven of these patients had a normal defaecation frequency and feeling of urgency after treatment. Similar results were reported at the same time by Weber et al. [12].

Biofeedback treatment involves teaching the patient how to relax their pelvic floor appropriately during defaecation straining. The biofeedback component consists of the patient viewing a pressure trace derived from a pressure catheter in the anal canal, or an electromyographic trace derived from electrodes placed on the perianal skin or a plug electrode. Alternatively a balloon may be inserted into the rectum and the patient asked to expel it using abdominal muscles while simultaneously relaxing the anal sphincter.

Although biofeedback treatment was initially proposed for patients thought to have pelvic floor incoordination alone, it has also been shown to be effective in patients with documented slow colonic transit combined with pelvic floor dysfunction. In some patients the treatment is useful in restoring bowel frequency and colonic transit time to normal, even if pelvic floor relaxation is initially normal [13].

The mechanism by which biofeedback treatment helps patients is likely to be complex and to differ in different types of patients. In some, correction of the pelvic floor abnormality may be the most important element of the treatment. In these patients pelvic floor contraction may not only inhibit rectal evacuation, but may promote retrograde peristalsis in the rectum and left colon. In others, the behavioural therapy may disinhibit the cerebral control of colonic motility. In yet others coming off laxatives and relearning a routine for defaecation, under supervision, may allow their normal bowel function to re-express itself.

Biofeedback combined with relaxation training or other psychotherapeutic techniques may be more successful than biofeedback alone [14]. Behavioural treatment depends on a good relationship between the therapist and the patient. In addition to relearning pelvic floor relaxation, patients also learn about appropriate use of their thoracic and abdominal muscles during straining. Many patients spontaneously talk about major personal concerns, including sexual problems, during biofeedback treatment. Although psychological therapy may well form a part of the treatment, patients find the physical therapy of biofeedback more acceptable than initial psychotherapy [15].

A large number of specialist centres have now reported their results using biofeedback treatment to treat intractable constipation [16]. In most series approximately 50 to 80 percent of patients are symptomatically improved. The benefit appears to be sustained in the long term [17].

A recent study followed up 100 patients who had been treated by biofeedback for idiopathic constipation more than 12 months previously [18]. Eighty seven patients were female. Their median age was 40 years and the mean duration of their constipation was 19 years. After a median follow-up of 23 months, 55 percent of patients felt they were still improved. There was a significant reduction in the need to strain (86% v 56%, pre v post, $p < 0.01$), abdominal pain ($p = 0.0004$), and oral laxative use (66% v 38%, $p < 0.01$). Spontaneous bowel frequency was improved by treatment. Patients with slow and normal transit, males and females, and those with and without pelvic floor contraction on straining, benefited equally from treatment.

Although apparently effective in many patients, there are few controlled studies of the effectiveness of this technique against placebo. Nonetheless, placebo responses are not believed to persist as long as the benefits which have been demonstrated with biofeedback and habit training.

Studies are needed to show whether this treatment results in improved patient quality of life.

Botulinum A toxin and puborectalis division

Botulinum A toxin has been used in the treatment of disorders of the ocular muscles such as blepharospasm and strabismus and also in torticollis. It is a neurotoxin produced by *Clostridium botulinum* which causes irreversible neuromuscular blockade and flaccid paralysis. Patients with inappropriate puborectalis contraction have been treated with injections into the muscle. The treatment is successful in decreasing the voluntary anal contraction pressure, the amount of straining and abdominal pain, but it does not improve patients bowel frequency and is no longer in use.

Surgical division of the puborectalis muscle has also been used to improve defaecation, but did not provide long term benefit.

Pelvic floor dysfunction and the results of colectomy

Biofeedback and other conservative treatments are adequate for most patients. Very rarely surgery is required. The traditional operation for patients with constipation and slow transit has been colectomy and ileorectal anastomosis. It has been postulated that inappropriate pelvic floor contraction is an adverse prognostic factor in patients with severe constipation being considered for a colectomy [19, 20]. Yet there is little or no evidence to support this. Wexner et al. [19] selected patients for colectomy on the basis of a slow intestinal transit time, measured with radioopaque markers, and the absence of inappropriate puborectalis contraction on cinedefaecography or electromyography. Most patients fared well. Similar findings were reported by Sunderland et al. [20] who investigated and treated patients according to a similar protocol. However, in both these studies follow-up was short; in studies with longer follow-up [21, 22] the outcome is more variable. In addition, no patients were operated on who had abnormal pelvic floor activity – they may have done as well if treated in the same way [22].

Other pelvic floor tests have been studied as potential predictors of outcome after colectomy for constipation. The presence of paradoxical pelvic floor contraction [22] or poor rectal emptying on proctography [23] preoperatively do not correlate with outcome. However, rectal balloon expulsion does appear to have some predictive value. Of 25 patients who were tested prior to a colectomy, 14 patients were not able to expel a balloon and all of these continued to experience pain and 8 continued to require laxatives [23]. Of the 11 patients who were able to expel a balloon, 6 continued to experience pain postoperatively and one still needed laxatives. Use of laxatives postoperatively may reflect abnormal rectal function and the need to strain excessively, or it may be a reflection of a psychological disturbance.

Conclusions

The symptom of impaired rectal evacuation represents a complex disorder encompassing a range of physical and psychological causes. Most patients can be symptomatically improved using behavioural techniques, with studies now showing evidence of long term benefit.

References

1. Preston DM, Lennard-Jones JE. Anismus in chronic constipation. *Dig Dis Sci* 1985; 30: 413-8.
2. Siproudhis L, Ropert A, Lucas J, Raoul JL, Heresbach D, Bretagne JF, Gosselin M. Defecatory disorders, anorectal and pelvic floor dysfunction: a polygamy? *Int J Colorectal Dis* 1992; 7: 102-7.
3. Drossman DA, Leserman J, Nachman G, Li Z, Gluck H, Toomey TC, Mitchell CM. Sexual and physical abuse in women with functional or organic gastrointestinal disorders. *Ann Inter Med* 1990; 113: 828-33.
4. Womack NR, Williams NS, Holmfield JHM, Morrison JFB, Simpkins KC. New method for the dynamic assessment of anorectal function in constipation. *Br J Surg* 1985; 72: 994-8.
5. Miller R, Duthie GS, Bartolo DCC, Roe AM, Locke-Edmunds J, Mortensen NJ. Anismus in patients with normal and slow transit constipation. *Br J Surg* 1991; 78: 690-2.
6. Wald A, Caruana BJ, Freimans MG, Bauman DH, Hinds JP. Contributions of evacuation proctography and anorectal manometry to evaluation of adults with constipation and defecatory difficulty. *Dig Dis Sci* 1990; 35: 481-7.

7. Jones PN, Lubowski DZ, Swash M, Henry MM. Is paradoxical contraction of the puborectalis muscle of functional importance? *Dis Col Rectum* 1987; 30: 667-70.
8. Johansson C, Nilsson BY, Mellgren A, Dolk A, Holmstrom B. Paradoxical sphincter reaction and associated colorectal disorders. *Int J Colorectal Dis* 1992; 7: 89-94.
9. Mathers SE, Kempster PA, Swash M, Lees AJ. Constipation and paradoxical puborectalis contraction in animus and Parkinson's disease: a dystonic phenomenon? *J Neurol Neurosurg Psychiatry* 1988; 51: 1503-7.
10. Mason HJ, Serrano-Ikkos E, Kamm MA. Women with idiopathic constipation have marked psychological morbidity, altered female self perception, and increased somatization compared with healthy women and Crohn's disease. *Gastroenterology* 1997; 112: A784.
11. Bleijenberg G, Kuijpers HC. Treatment of spastic pelvic floor syndrome with biofeedback. *Dis Col Rectum* 1987; 30: 108-11.
12. Weber J, Ducrotte P, Touchais JY, Roussignol C, Denis P. Biofeedback training for constipation in adults and children. *Dis Col Rectum* 1987; 30: 844-6.
13. Koutsomanis D, Lennard-Jones JE, Kamm MA. Prospective study of biofeedback treatment for patients with slow and normal transit constipation. *Eur J Gastro Hepatol* 1994; 6: 131-7.
14. Turnbull GK, Ritvo PG. Anal sphincter biofeedback relaxation treatment for women with intractable constipation symptoms. *Dis Col Rectum* 1992; 35: 530-6.
15. Denis P. Biofeedback for constipation. In: Kamm MA, Lennard-Jones JE, eds. *Constipation*. Petersfield: Wrightson Biomedical Publishing, 1994: 349-53.
16. Kamm MA. Motility and functional diseases of the large intestine. *Current Op Gastroenterol* 1993; 9: 11-8.
17. Koutsomanis D, Lennard-Jones JE, Roy AJ, Kamm MA. Controlled randomised trial of biofeedback versus muscle training alone for intractable constipation. *Gut* 1995; 37: 95-9.
18. Chiotakakou-Faliakou E, Kamm MA, Roy AJ, Storrie JB, Turner IC. Biofeedback provides long term benefit for patients with intractable slow and normal transit constipation. *Gastroenterology* 1997; 112: A712.
19. Wexner SD, Daniel N, Jagelman DG. Colectomy for constipation: physiological investigation is the key to success. *Dis Col Rectum* 1991; 34: 851-6.
20. Sunderland GT, Poon FW, Lauder J, Finlay IG. Videoproctography in selecting patients with constipation for colectomy. *Dis Col Rectum* 1992; 35: 235-7.
21. Leon SH, Krishnamurthy S, Schuffler MD. Subtotal colectomy for severe idiopathic constipation. *Dig Dis Sci* 1987; 32: 1249-53.
22. Kamm MA, Hawley PR, Lennard-Jones JE. Outcome of colectomy for severe idiopathic constipation. *Gut* 1988; 29: 969-73.
23. Van der Sijp JRM, Kamm MA, Lennard-Jones JE. Age of onset and rectal emptying: predicting outcome of colectomy for severe idiopathic constipation. *Int J Colorectal Dis* 1992; 7: 35-7.

Achevé d'imprimer par Corlet, Imprimeur, S.A.
14110 Condé-sur-Noireau (France)
N° d'Imprimeur : 26606 - Dépôt légal : octobre 1997

Imprimé en C.E.E.